The Delicious Mediterranean Dessert Recipe Book

Easy and Tasty Dessert Recipes to Boost Your Meals and Satisfy Your Taste

Bill Gibbs

Table of contents

Hemp Cocoa Cookies

Prep time: 30 minutes I **Cooking time:** 0 minutes I
Servings: 6

Ingredients:

- 1 cup almonds, soaked overnight and drained
- 2 tablespoons cocoa powder
- 1 tablespoon coconut sugar
- ½ cup hemp seeds
- ¼ cup coconut, shredded
- ½ cup water

Directions:

1. In your food processor, combine the almonds with the cocoa powder and the other ingredients, pulse well, press this on a lined baking sheet, keep in the fridge for 30 minutes, slice and serve.

Nutrition info per serving: calories 270, fat 12.6, fiber 3, carbs 7.7, protein 7

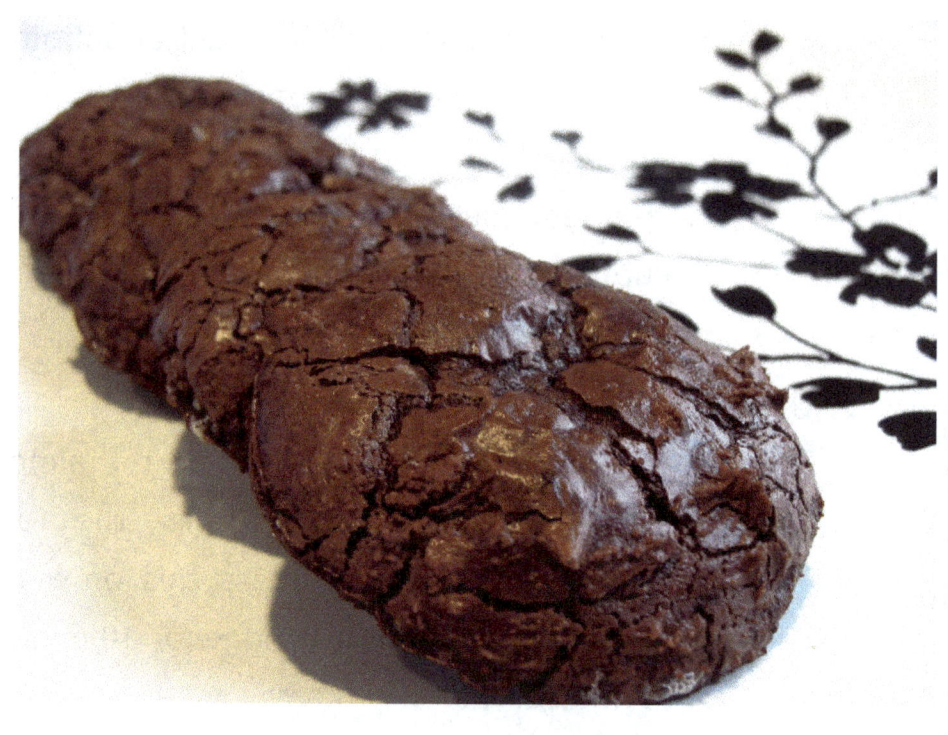

Pomegranate Bowls

Prep time: 2 hours I **Cooking time:** 0 minutes I
Servings: 4

Ingredients:

- ½ cup coconut cream
- 1 teaspoon vanilla extract
- 1 cup almonds, chopped
- 1 cup pomegranate seeds
- 1 tablespoon coconut sugar

Directions:

1. In a bowl, combine the almonds with the cream and the other ingredients, toss, divide into small bowls and serve.

Nutrition info per serving: calories 258, fat 19, fiber 3.9, carbs 17.6, protein 6.2

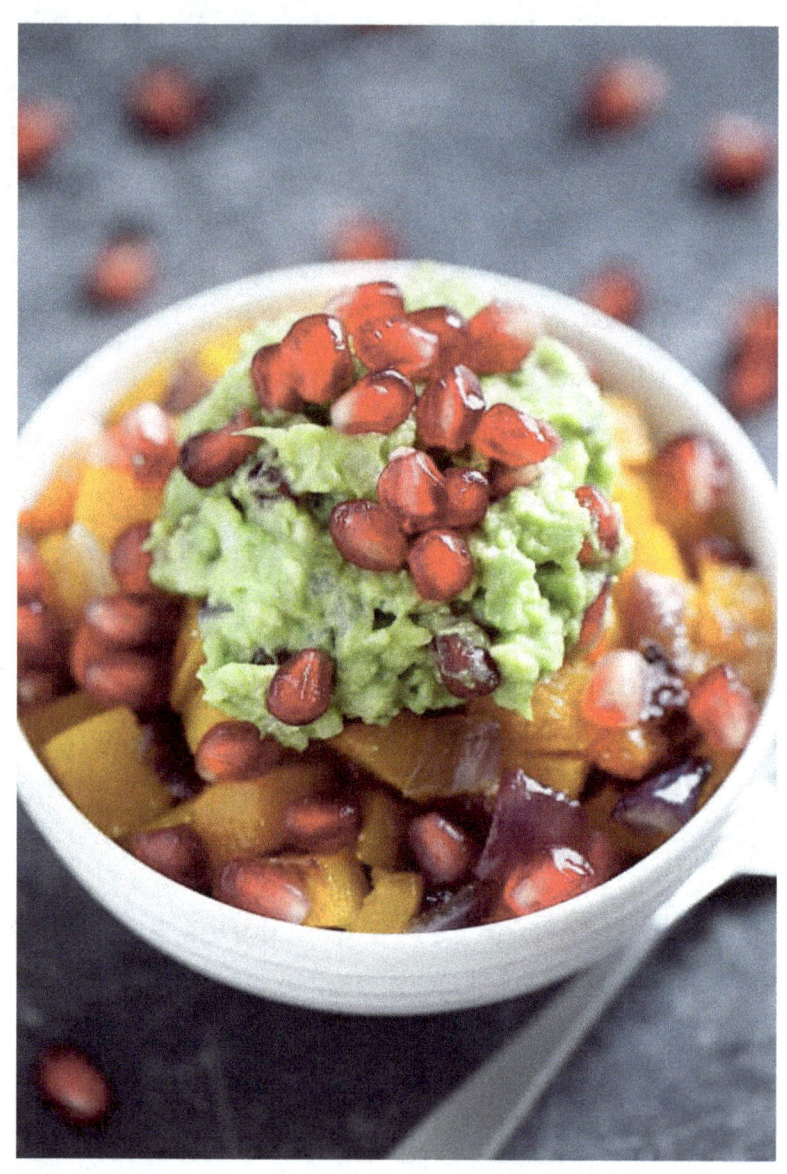

Chia and Blackberries Cream

Prep time: 10 minutes I **Cooking time:** 0 minutes I
Servings: 6

Ingredients:

- 2 cups coconut cream
- 2/3 cup coconut sugar
- ½ cup blackberries
- 1 cup almond milk
- 3 tablespoons chia seeds, ground
- ½ teaspoon vanilla extract

Directions:

1. In a bowl, combine the cream with the chia seeds and the other ingredients, whisk well, divide into small bowls, leave aside for 10 minutes and serve.

Nutrition info per serving: calories 295, fat 29.2, fiber 3.3, carbs 9.6, protein 3.3

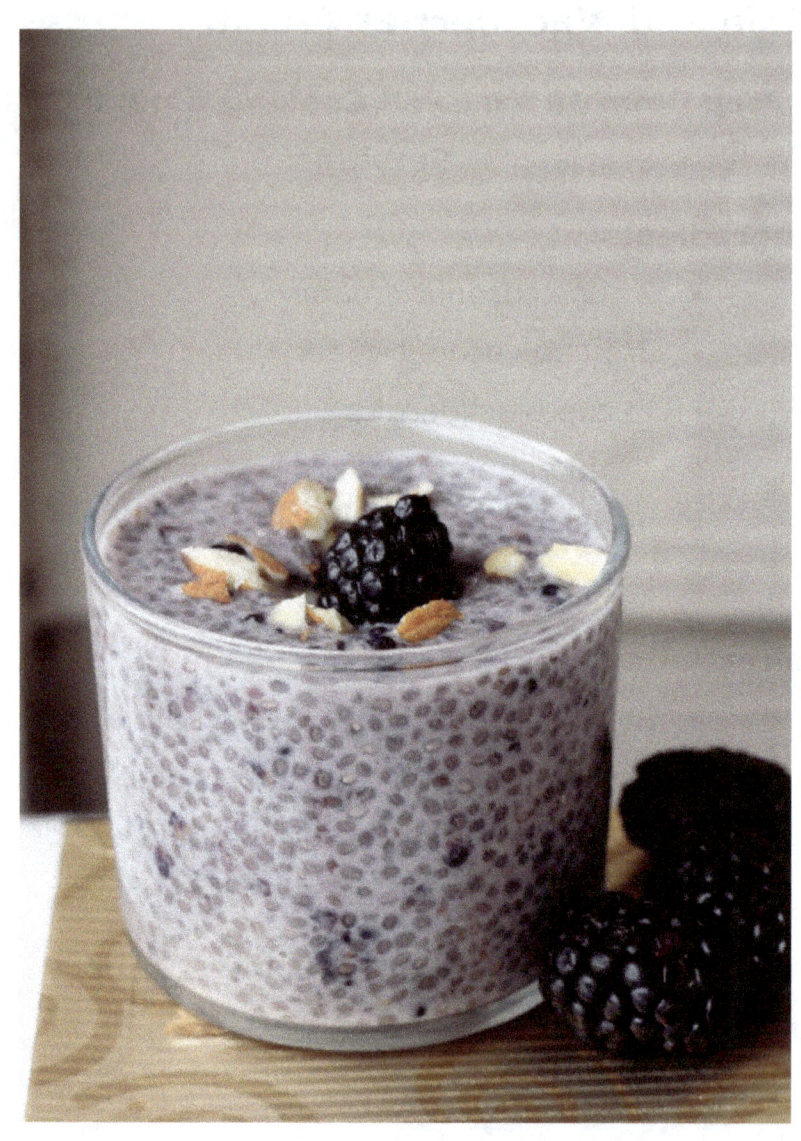

Lime Berries Salad

Prep time: 5 minutes I **Cooking time:** 0 minutes I
Servings: 4

Ingredients:

- 1 cup blackberries
- 1 cup blueberries
- 1 tablespoon lime juice
- 1 cup strawberries, halved
- 1 tablespoon coconut sugar
- ½ teaspoon ginger powder
- ½ teaspoon vanilla extract

Directions:

1. In a bowl, combine the blackberries with the blueberries and the other ingredients, toss and serve.

Nutrition info per serving: calories 77, fat 0.4, fiber 3.6, carbs 17.4, protein 1.3

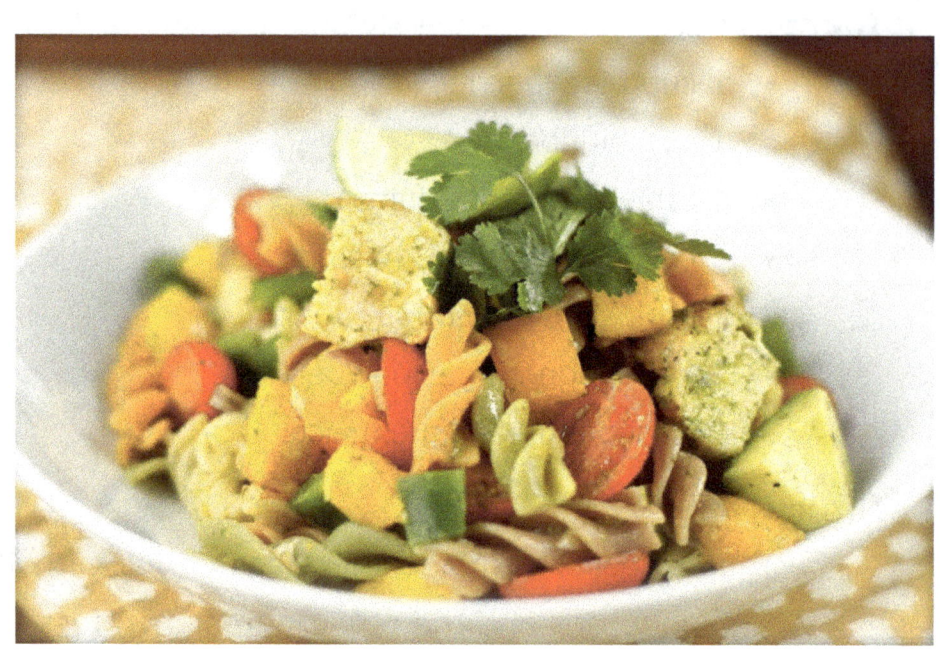

Grapefruit Cream

Prep time: 10 minutes I **Cooking time:** 10 minutes I
Servings: 4

Ingredients:

- 1 cup coconut milk
- 2 tablespoons coconut sugar
- ½ cup coconut cream
- 1 teaspoon vanilla extract
- 4 grapefruits, peeled and roughly chopped

Directions:

1. In a pan, combine the milk with the grapefruits and the other ingredients, whisk, bring to a simmer and cook over medium heat for 10 minutes.
2. Blend using an immersion blender, divide into bowls and serve cold.

Nutrition info per serving: calories 298, fat 21.6, carbs 3.4, fiber 25, protein 3.4

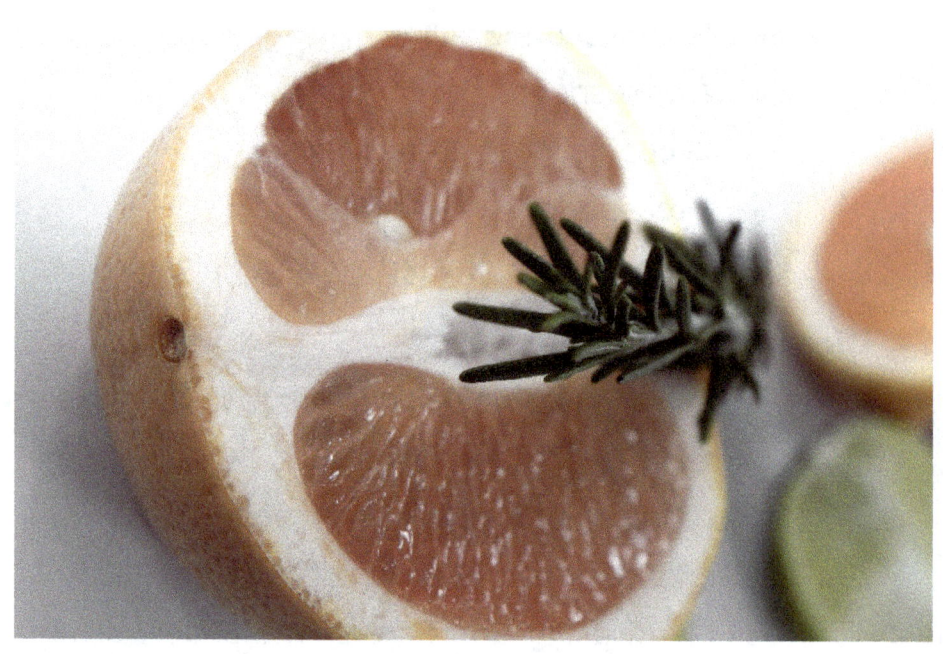

Mango Mix

Prep time: 10 minutes I **Cooking time:** 0 minutes I
Servings: 4

Ingredients:

- 2 bananas, peeled and sliced
- 2 mangoes, peeled and cubed
- 1 tablespoon walnuts, chopped
- 1 tablespoon lime juice

Directions:

1. In a bowl, combine the bananas with the mangoes and the other ingredients, toss and serve.

Nutrition info per serving: calories 165, fat 2, fiber 4.4, carbs 38.8, protein 2.5

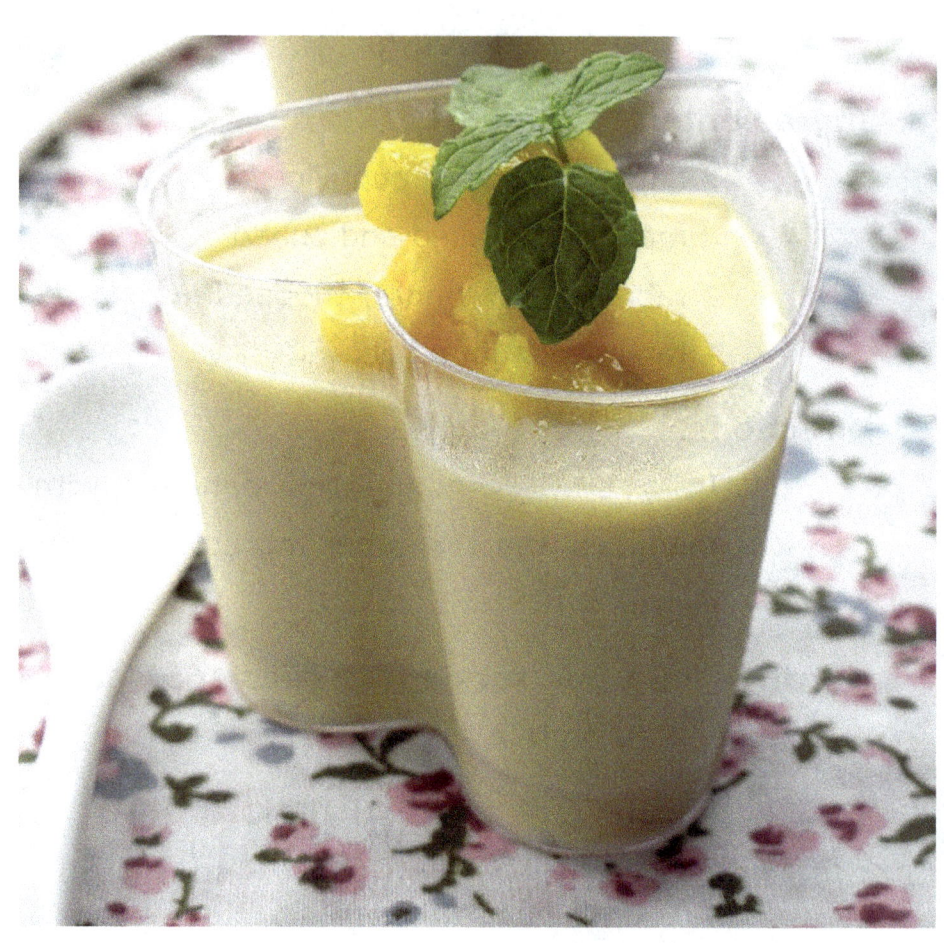

Mango Cream

Prep time: 2 hours I **Cooking time:** 0 minutes I
Servings: 6

Ingredients:

- 1 watermelon, peeled and cubed
- 1 teaspoon vanilla extract
- ½ teaspoon cinnamon powder
- 2 mangoes, peeled and cubed

Directions:

1. In a blender, combine the watermelon with the mango and the other ingredients, pulse well, divide into bowls and keep in the fridge for 2 hours before serving.

Nutrition info per serving: calories 75, fat 0.5, fiber 1.9, carbs 18.4, protein 1

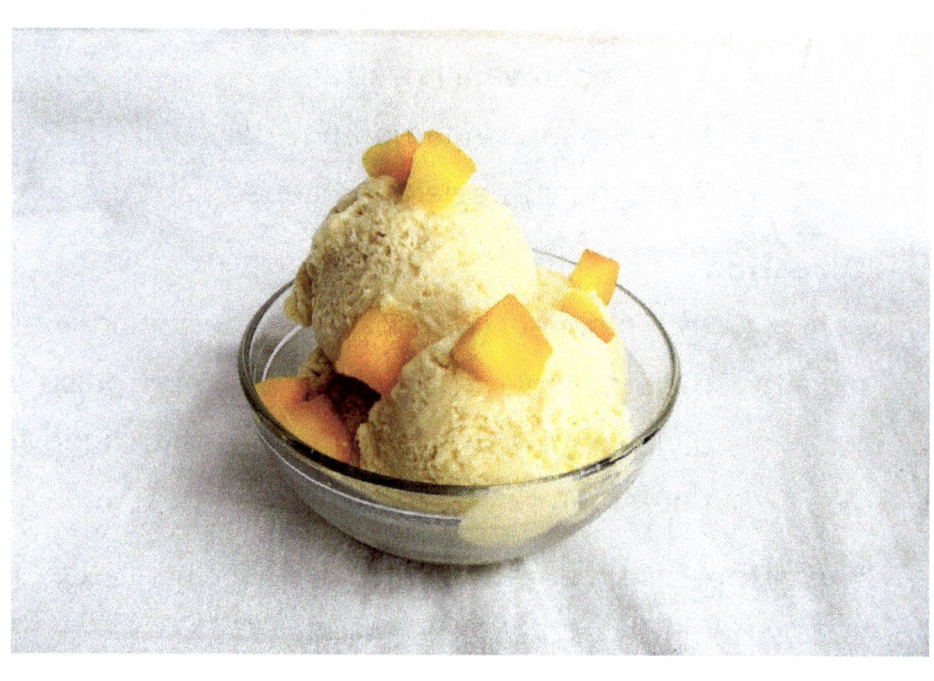

Cocoa Dates

Prep time: 10 minutes I **Cooking time:** 0 minutes I
Servings: 4

Ingredients:

- 1 cup dates, chopped
- 2 bananas, peeled and sliced
- 1 cup almond milk
- 2 tablespoons cocoa powder
- 1 tablespoon honey

Directions:

1. In a bowl, combine the dates with the bananas and the other ingredients, toss and serve cold.

Nutrition info per serving: calories 338, fat 15, fiber 7.2, carbs 56, protein 3.6

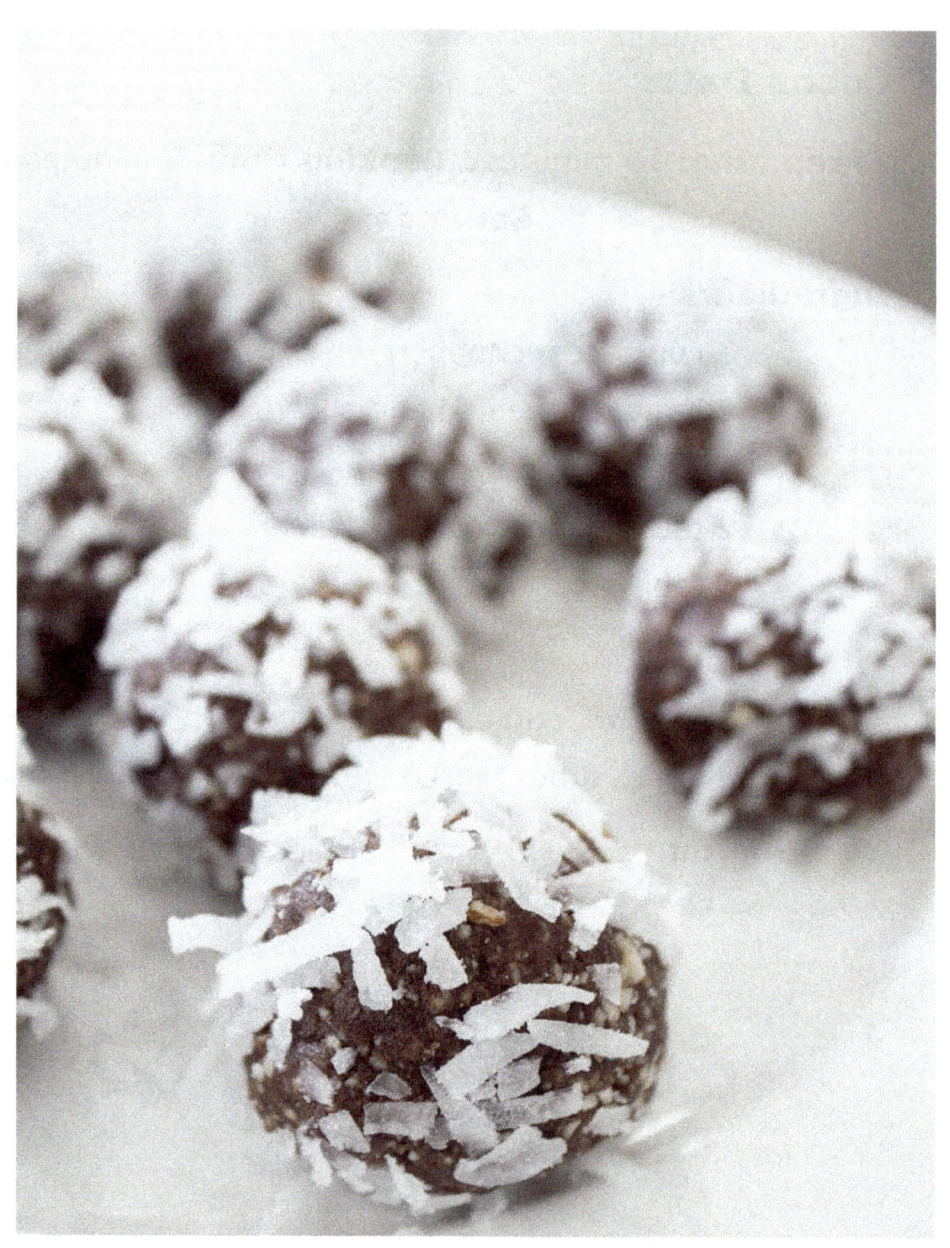

Creamy Apple

Prep time: 10 minutes I **Cooking time:** 0 minutes I
Servings: 2

Ingredients:

- 2 big green apples, cored and roughly cubed
- 1 tablespoon honey
- 1 cup coconut cream
- 1 teaspoon cinnamon powder

Directions:

1. In a bowl, combine the apples with the cream and the other ingredients, toss and serve.

Nutrition info per serving: calories 100, fat 1, fiber 4, carbs 12, protein 4

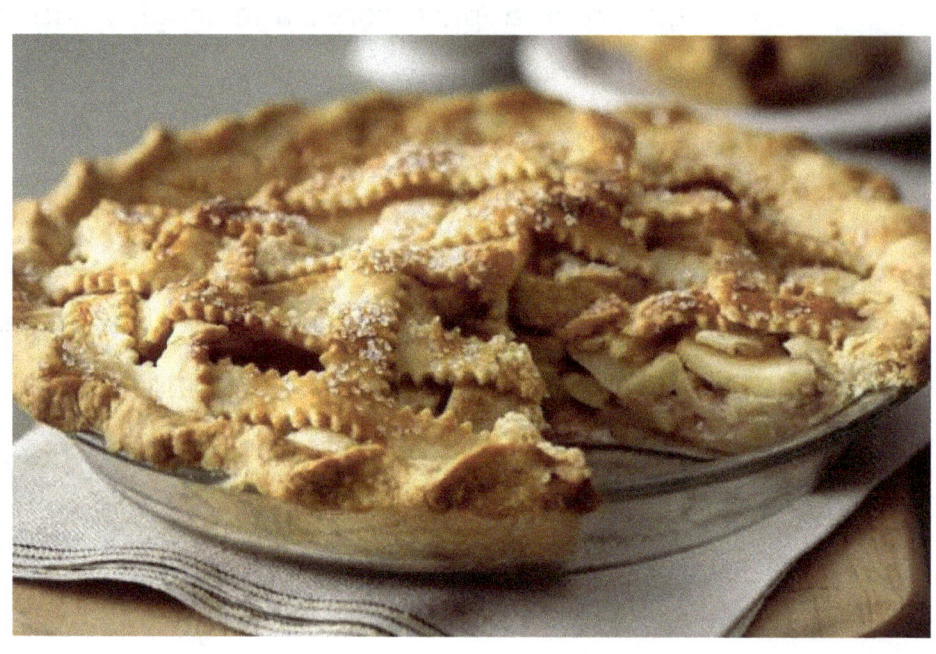

Nuts Cream

Prep time: 10 minutes I **Cooking time:** 20 minutes I
Servings: 6

Ingredients:

- 1 cup pineapple, peeled and cubed
- ½ cup walnuts, chopped
- 1 tablespoon honey
- 1 cup coconut cream
- 1 egg, whisked
- ¼ cup coconut oil, melted

Directions:

1. In a blender, combine the pineapple with the walnuts and the other ingredients, pulse well, divide into 6 ramekins and bake at 370 degrees F for 20 minutes.
2. Serve cold.

Nutrition info per serving: calories 200, fat 3, fiber 4, carbs 12, protein 8

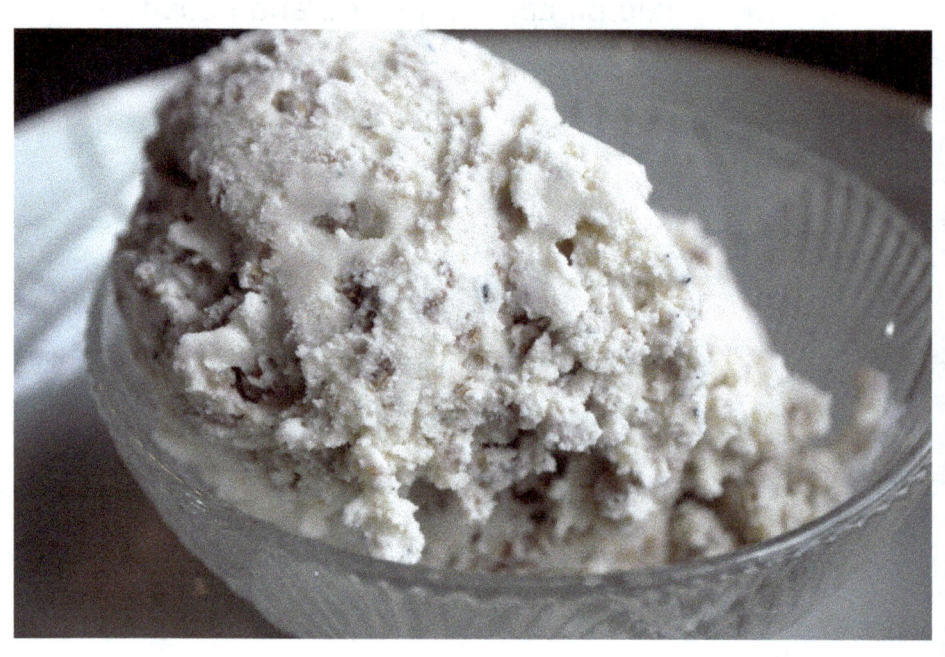

Maple Bars

Prep time: 10 minutes I **Cooking time:** 25 minutes I
Servings: 6

Ingredients:

- ½ cup coconut cream
- 1 cup apples, peeled, cored and chopped
- ½ cup maple syrup
- 1 teaspoon vanilla extract
- ½ cup almond flour
- 2 eggs, whisked
- 1 teaspoon baking powder

Directions:

1. In a blender, combine the cream with the apples and the other ingredients and pulse well.
2. Pour this into a baking dish lined with parchment paper, bake in the oven at 370 degrees F for 25 minutes, cool down, cut into bars and serve.

Nutrition info per serving: calories 200, fat 3, fiber 4, carbs 12, protein 11

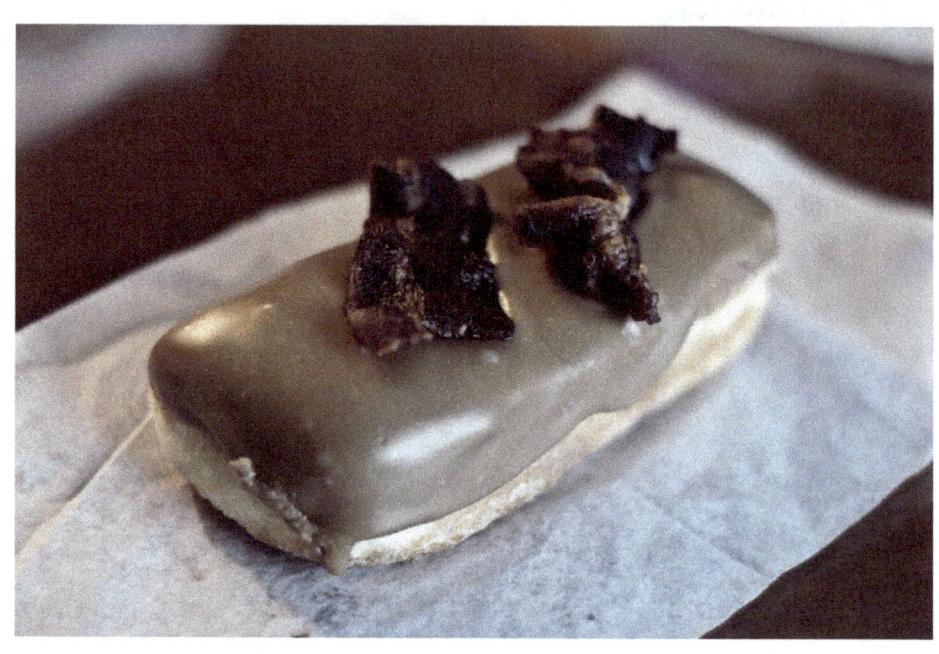

Avocado Salad

Prep time: 10 minutes I **Cooking time:** 0 minutes I
Servings: 6

Ingredients:

- 3 oranges, peeled and cut into segments
- 1 avocado, peeled, pitted and cubed
- 3 tablespoons raw honey
- ½ teaspoon vanilla extract
- 1 teaspoon orange zest, grated

Directions:

1. In a bowl, combine the oranges with the avocado and the other ingredients, toss and serve.

Nutrition info per serving: calories 211, fat 3, fiber 4, carbs 8, protein 7

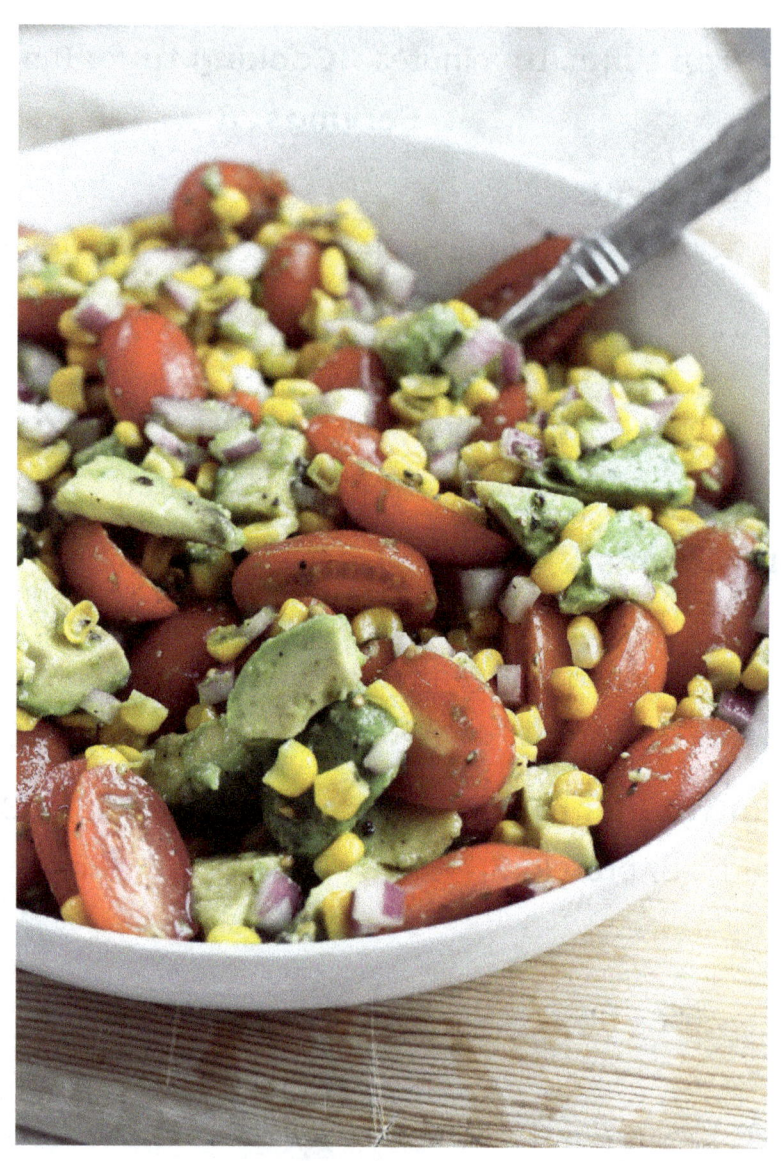

Ginger Apples

Prep time: 10 minutes I **Cooking time:** 30 minutes I
Servings: 4

Ingredients:

- 2 apples, cored and halved
- 1 tablespoon ginger, grated
- 1 tablespoon turmeric powder
- ¼ cup raw honey
- 1 tablespoon ginger, grated

Directions:

1. Arrange the apples in a baking dish, add the ginger and the other ingredients, and bake at 390 degrees F for 30 minutes.
2. Divide the apples mix between dessert plates and serve.

Nutrition info per serving: calories 90, fat 2, fiber 1, carbs 2, protein 5

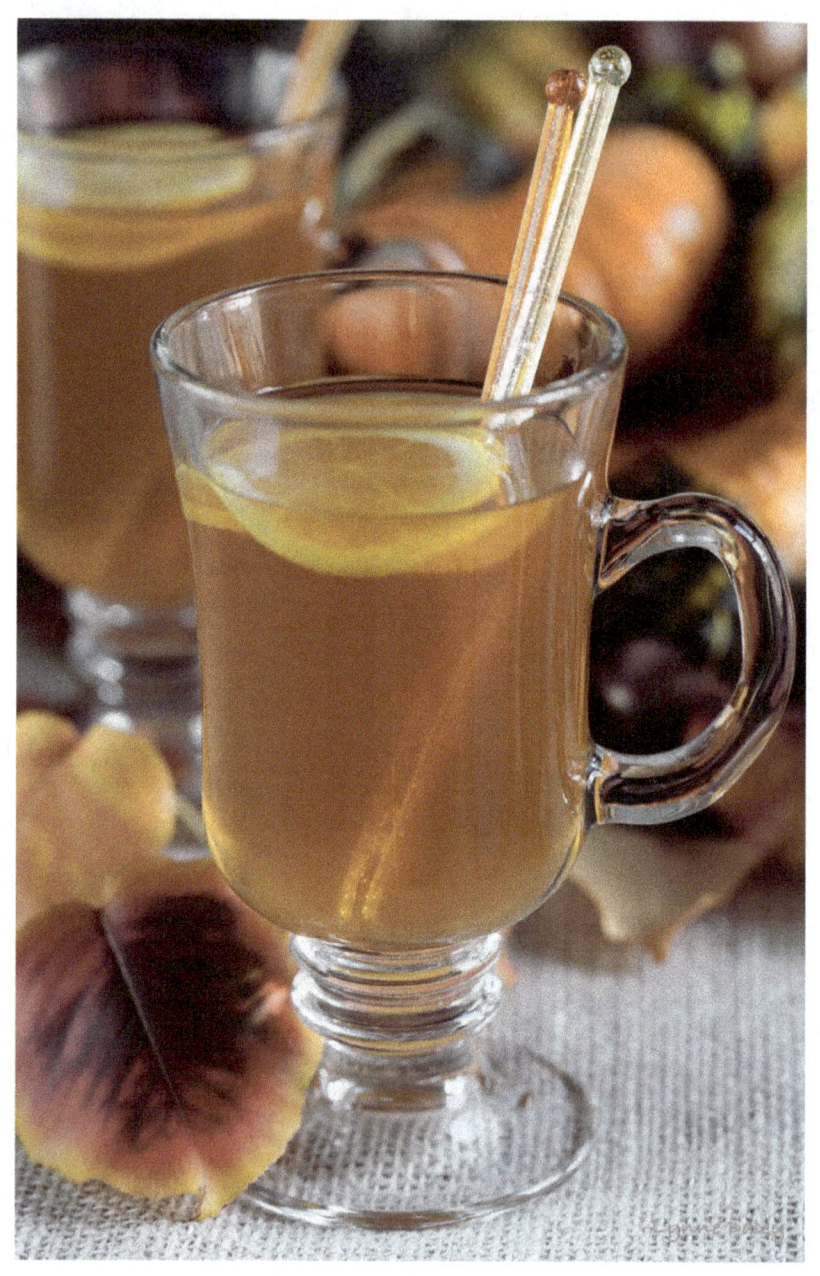

Watermelon Cream

Prep time: 2 hours I **Cooking time:** 0 minutes I
Servings: 4

Ingredients:

- 2 cups coconut cream
- 1 watermelon, peeled and chopped
- 2 avocados, peeled, pitted and chopped
- 1 tablespoon honey
- 2 teaspoons lemon juice

Directions:

1. In a blender, combine the watermelon with the cream and the other ingredients, pulse well, divide into bowls and keep in the fridge for 2 hours before serving.

Nutrition info per serving: calories 121, fat 2, fiber 2, carbs 6, protein 5

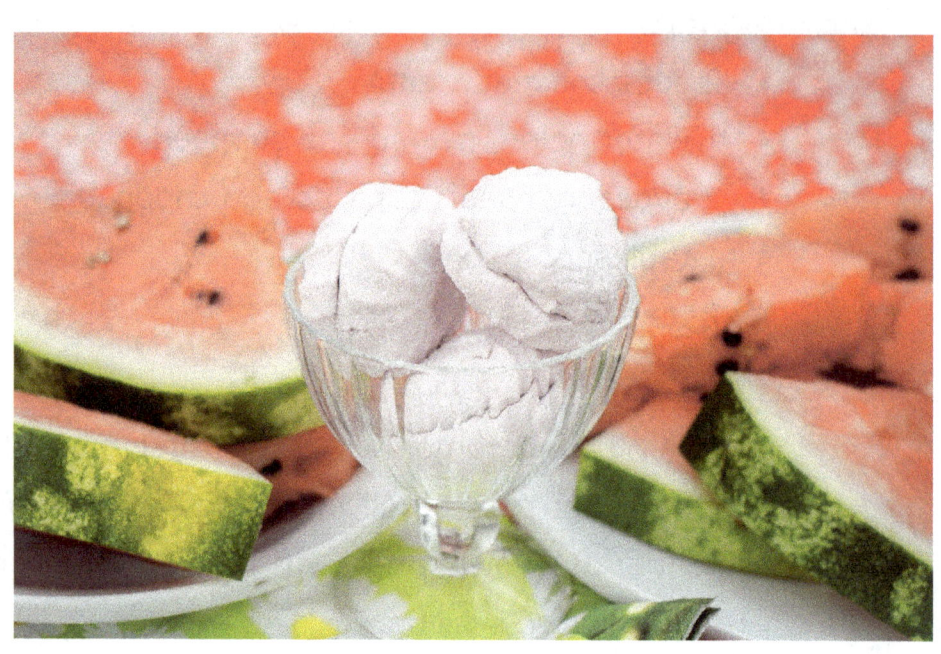

Honey Berry Sorbet

Prep time: 2 hours I **Cooking time:** 0 minutes I
Servings: 6

Ingredients:

- 1 pound strawberries, halved and frozen
- 1 cup orange juice
- 1 tablespoon orange zest, grated
- 1 tablespoon honey

Directions:

1. In a blender, combine the strawberries with the orange zest and the other ingredients, pulse well, divide into bowls and keep in the freezer for 2 hours before serving.

Nutrition info per serving: calories 121, fat 1, fiber 2, carbs 2, protein 4

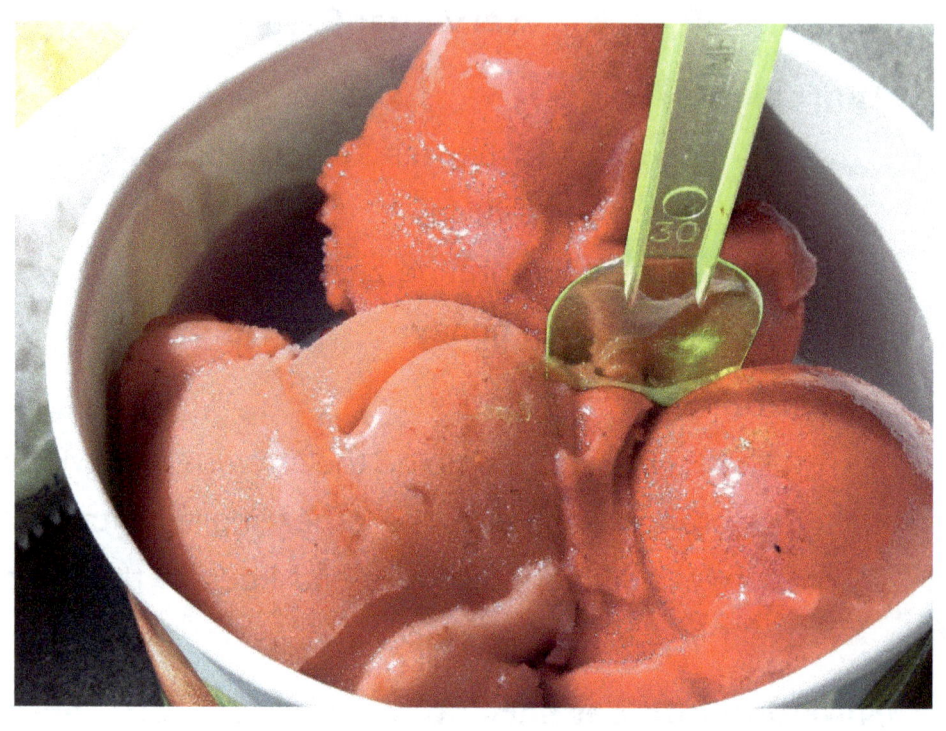

Lemony Mix

Prep time: 10 minutes I **Cooking time:** 0 minutes I
Servings: 4

Ingredients:

- 2 tablespoons almonds, chopped
- 1 tablespoon walnuts, chopped
- 2 cups pineapple, peeled and roughly cubed
- 1 tablespoon lemon juice
- Zest of 1 lemon, grated
- ½ teaspoon vanilla extract
- A pinch of cinnamon powder

Directions:

1. In a bowl, combine the pineapple with the nuts and the other ingredients, toss and serve.

Nutrition info per serving: calories 215, fat 3, fiber 4, carbs 12, protein 8

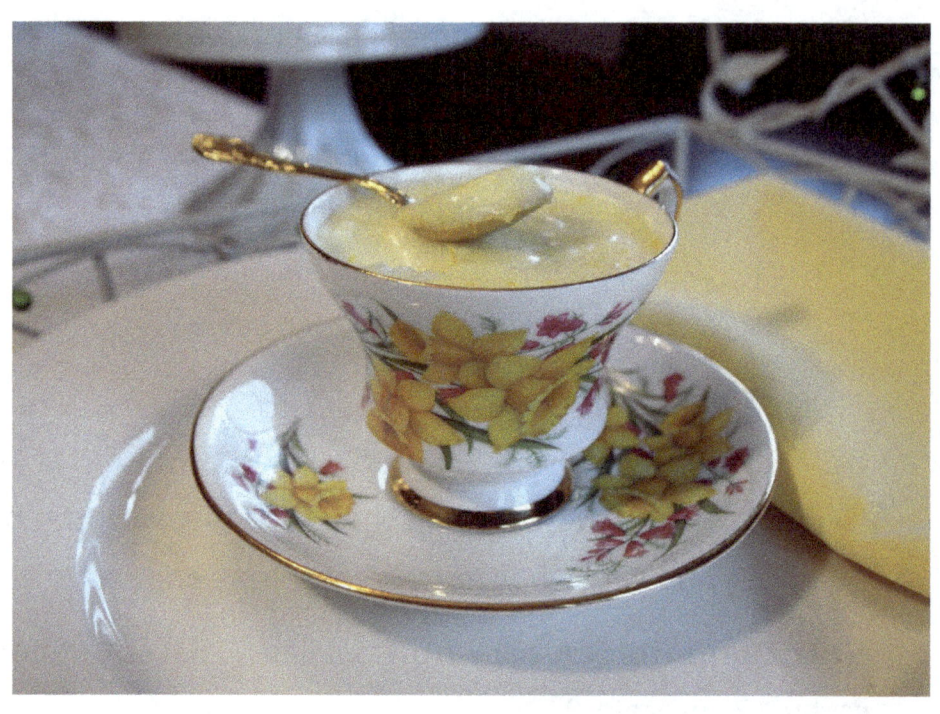

Cardamom Quinoa Pudding

Prep time: 30 minutes I **Cooking time:** 0 minutes I
Servings: 4

Ingredients:

- 2 cups almond milk
- 2 tablespoon honey
- 1 cup quinoa, cooked
- A pinch of cardamom powder
- 1 tablespoon lemon zest, grated

Directions:

1. In a bowl, mix the quinoa with the almond milk
   and the other ingredients, toss, leave aside for
   30 minutes, divide into small bowls and serve.

Nutrition info per serving: calories 199, fat 2, fiber 3,
carbs 7, protein 5

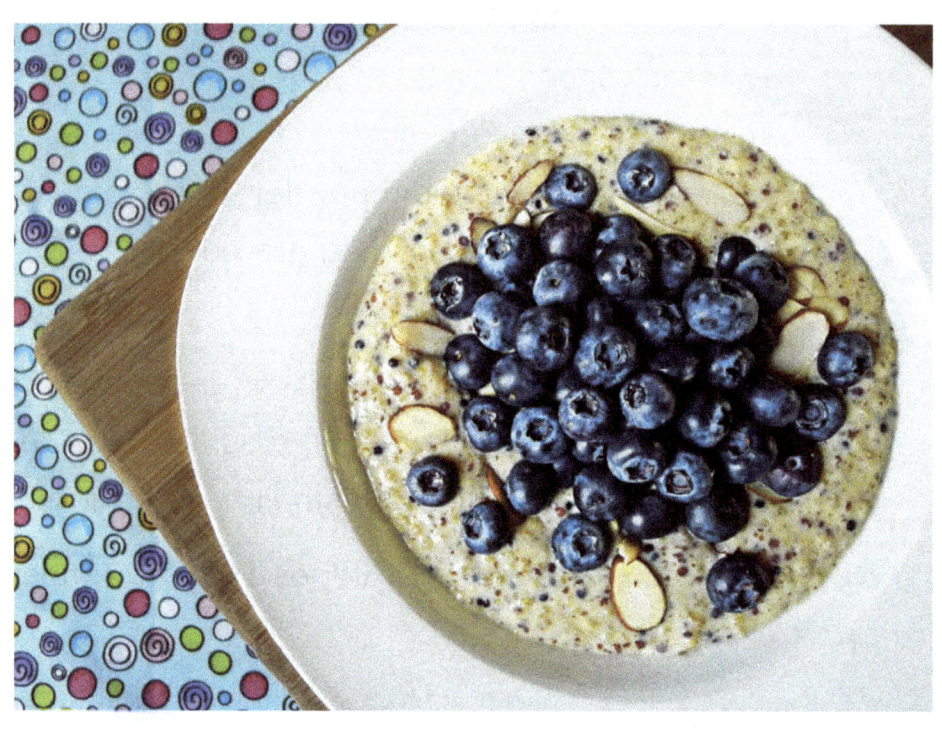

Orange Mango Smoothie

Prep time: 10 minutes I **Cooking time:** 0 minutes I
Servings: 2

Ingredients:

- 2 cups mango, peeled and c hopped
- 1 cup orange juice
- 1 tablespoon ginger, grated
- 1 teaspoon turmeric powder

Directions:

1. In your blender, combine the mango with the juice and the other ingredients, pulse well, divide into 2 glasses and serve cold.

Nutrition info per serving: calories 100, fat 1, fiber 2, carbs 4, protein 5

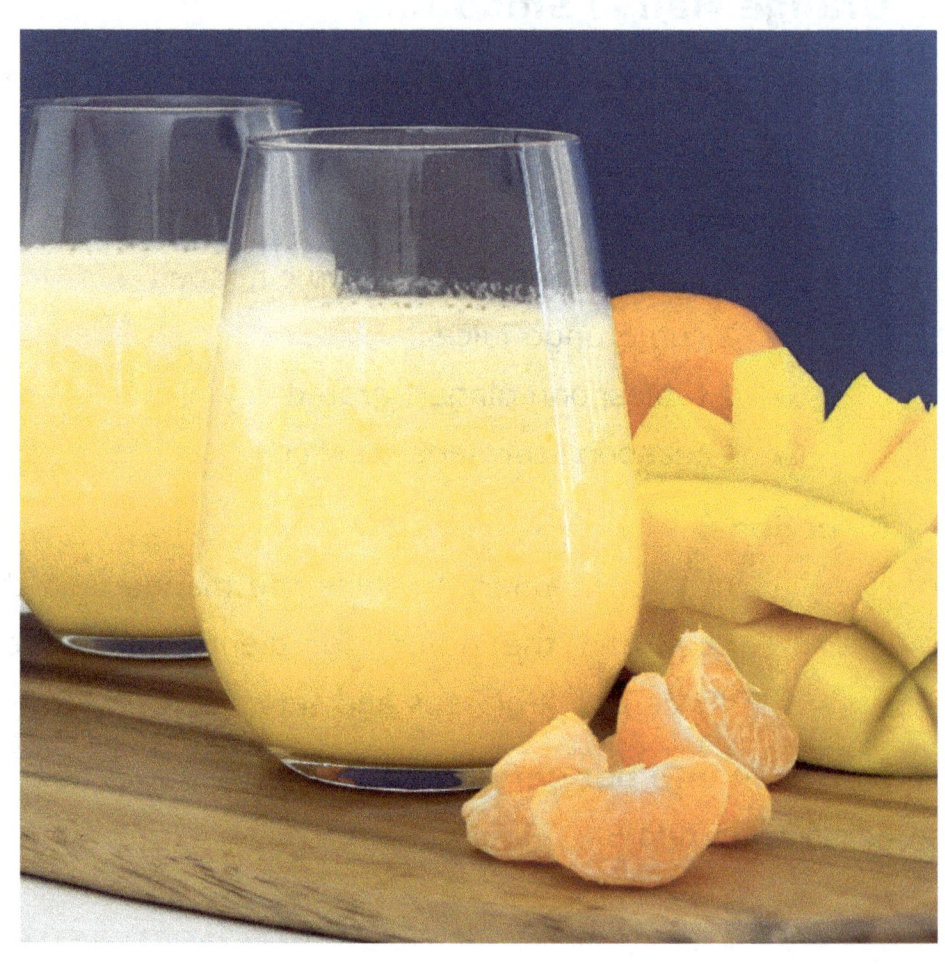

Chocolate Cream

Prep time: 2 hours I **Cooking time:** 0 minutes I
Servings: 4

Ingredients:

- 2 cups coconut milk
- 2 tablespoons ginger, grated
- 2 tablespoons honey
- 1 cup dark chocolate, chopped and melted
- ½ teaspoon cinnamon powder
- 1 teaspoon vanilla extract

Directions:

1. In a blender, combine the coconut milk with the ginger and the other ingredients, pulse well, divide into bowls and keep in the fridge for 2 hours before serving.

Nutrition info per serving: calories 200, fat 3, fiber 5, carbs 12, protein 7

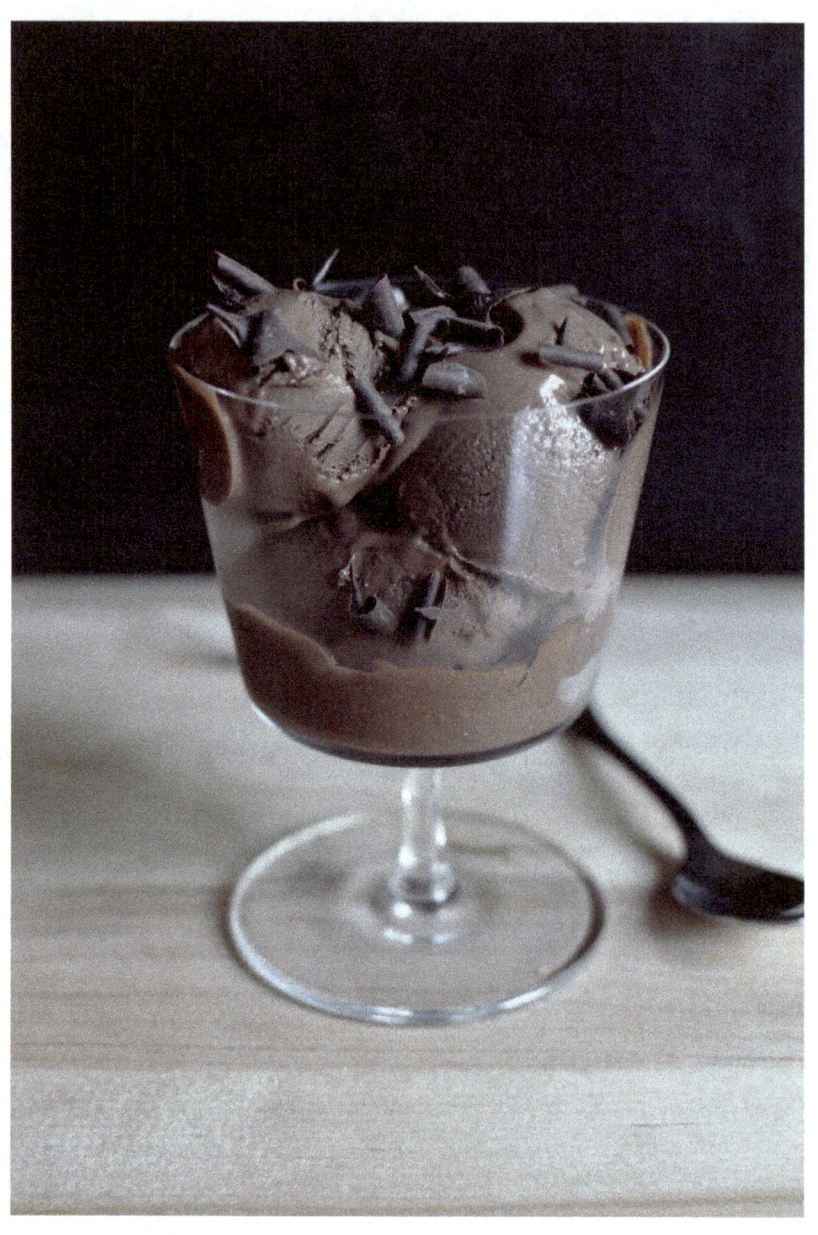

Buttery Avocado Mix

Prep time: 10 minutes I **Cooking time:** 0 minutes I
Servings: 4

Ingredients:

- 2 avocados, peeled, pitted and cut into wedges
- 1 teaspoon cardamom, ground
- ½ cup coconut butter
- 1 cup coconut cream
- 1 teaspoon vanilla extract

Directions:

1. In your food processor, combine the avocados with the cream and the other ingredients, pulse well, divide into bowls and serve cold.

Nutrition info per serving: calories 211, fat 2, fiber 4, carbs 11, protein 7

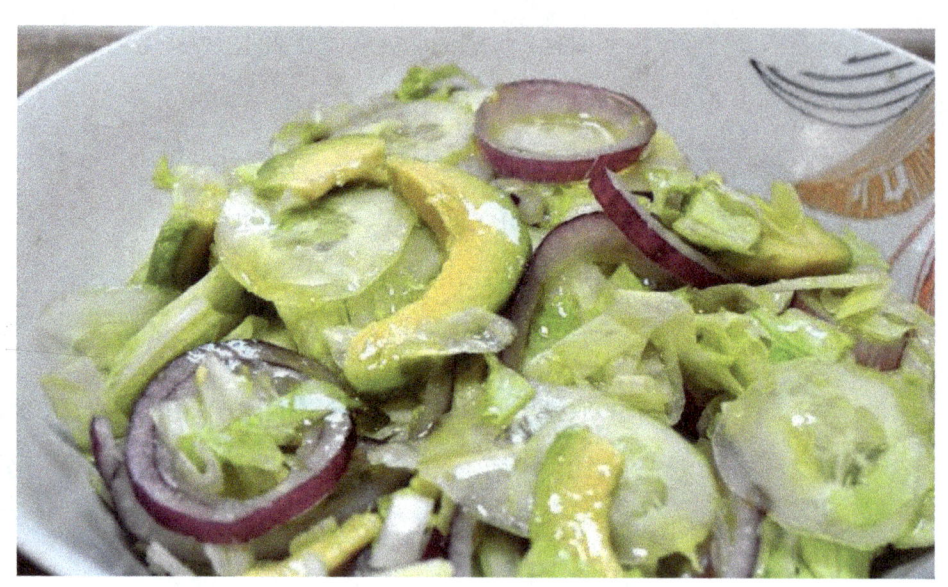

Baked Strawberries

Prep time: 10 minutes I **Cooking time:** 20 minutes I
Servings: 4

Ingredients:

- 1 pound strawberries, halved
- 2 tablespoons almonds, chopped
- 2 tablespoons avocado oil
- 2 tablespoons lime juice
- 1 teaspoon vanilla extract
- 1 teaspoon honey

Directions:

1. Arrange the strawberries on a baking sheet lined with parchment paper, add the almonds and the other ingredients, toss and bake at 390 degrees F for 20 minutes.
2. Divide the strawberries mix into bowls and serve.

Nutrition info per serving: calories 220, fat 2, fiber 3, carbs 8, protein 2

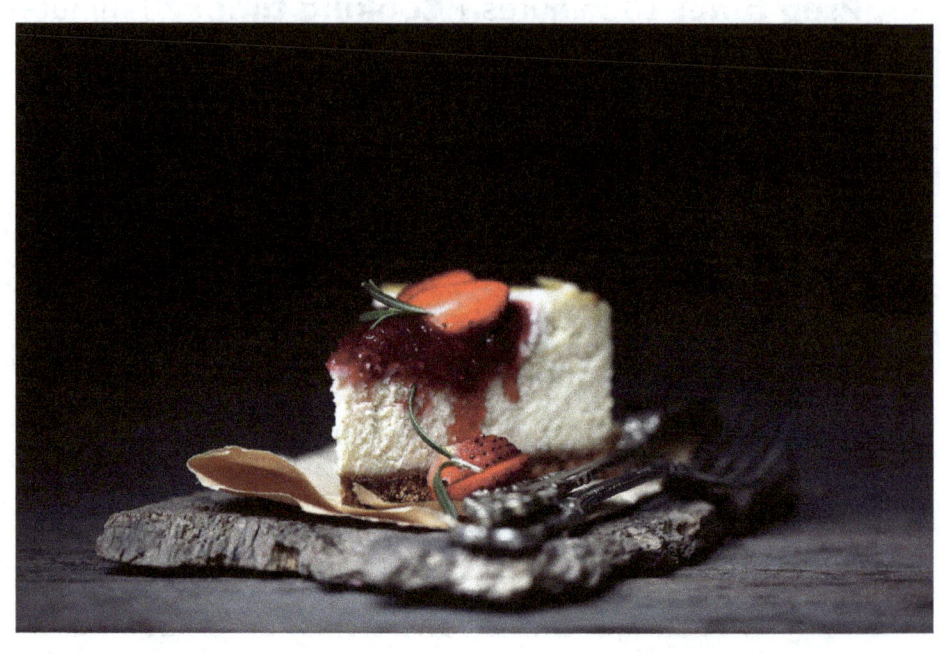

Apple Compote

Prep time: 10 minutes I **Cooking time:** 20 minutes I

Servings: 4

Ingredients:

- Juice of 1 lime
- 1 pound apples, cored and cut into wedges
- 1 tablespoon honey
- 1 and ½ cups water

Directions:

1. In a pan, combine the apples with the lime juice and the other ingredients, toss, bring to a simmer and cook over medium heat fro 20 minutes.
2. Divide the mix into bowls and serve cold.

Nutrition info per serving: calories 108, fat 1, fiber 2, carbs 4, protein 7

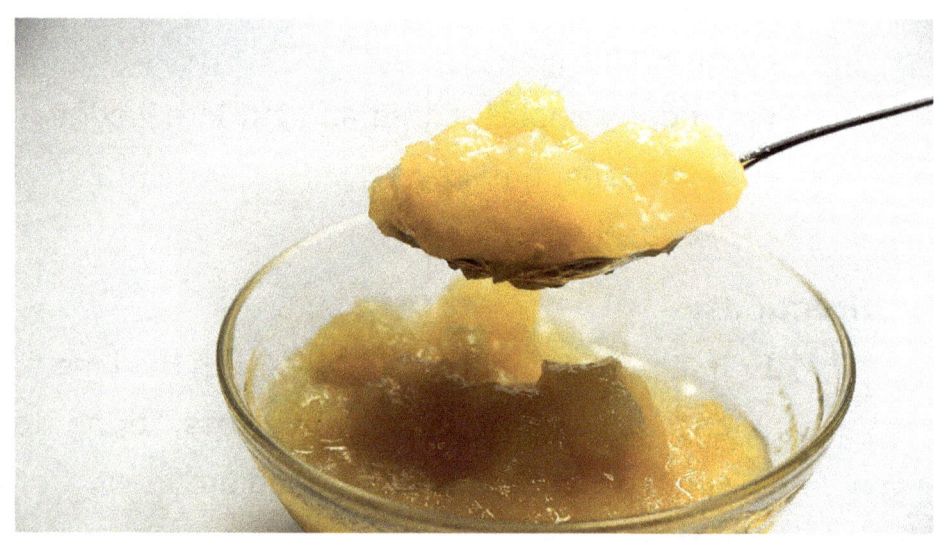

Vanilla Honey Berries

Prep time: 10 minutes I **Cooking time:** 0 minutes I
Servings: 4

Ingredients:

- 1 cup blackberries
- 1 cup blueberries
- 2 teaspoons lime zest, grated
- 1 tablespoon raw honey
- ½ teaspoon vanilla extract
- 1 cup almond milk

Directions:

1. In your blender, combine the berries with the
   lime zest and the other ingredients, pulse well,
   divide into bowls and serve.

Nutrition info per serving: calories 217, fat 7, fiber 8,
carbs 10, protein 8

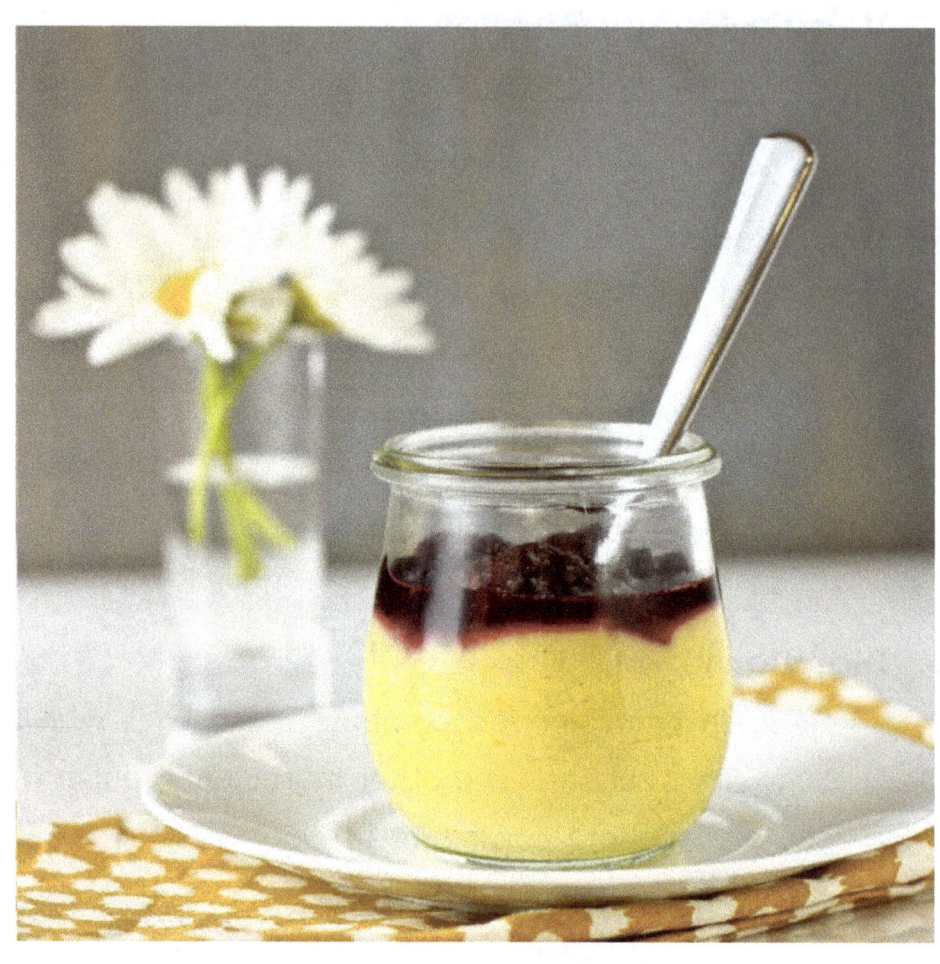

Maple Coconut Mix

Prep time: 10 minutes I **Cooking time:** 15 minutes I
Servings: 4

Ingredients:

- 2 cups coconut milk
- 1 cup strawberries
- ¼ teaspoon vanilla extract
- 1/3 cup pure maple syrup

Directions:

1. In a small pot, combine the coconut milk with the berries and the other ingredients, toss, cook over medium heat for 15 minutes, divide into bowls and serve cold.

Nutrition info per serving: calories 176, fat 4, fiber 2, carbs 7, protein 6

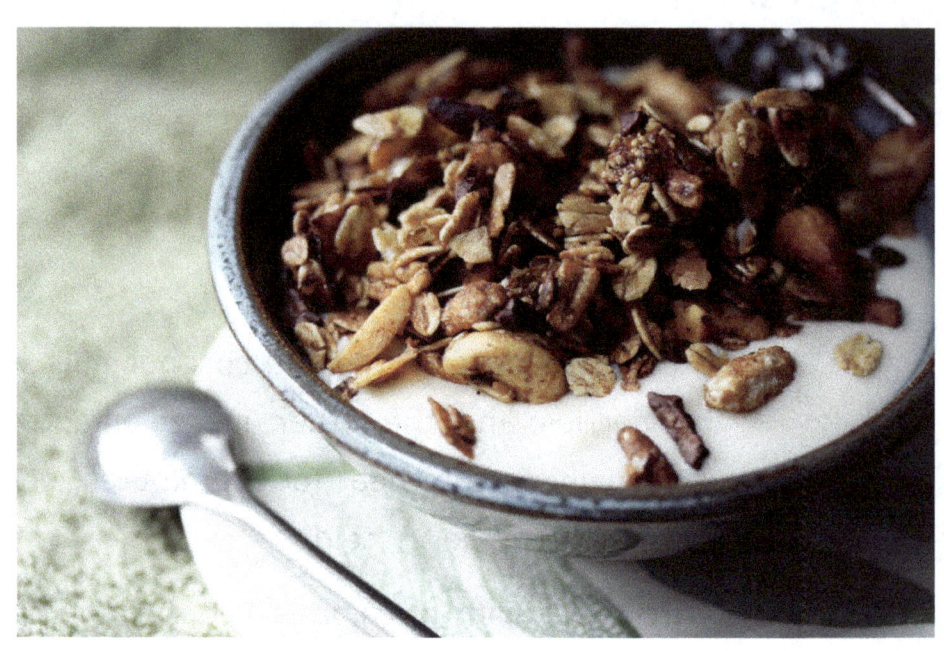

Papaya Bowls

Prep time: 4 minutes I **Cooking time:** 0 minutes I
Servings: 4

Ingredients:

- 1 cup papaya, roughly cubed
- ½ teaspoon vanilla extract
- 2 tablespoons almonds, chopped
- 1 tablespoon walnuts, chopped
- 2 tablespoons lemon juice

Directions:

1. In a bowl, combine the papaya with the other ingredients, toss, divide into smaller bowls and serve.

Nutrition info per serving: calories 140, fat 1, fiber 2, carbs 3, protein 5

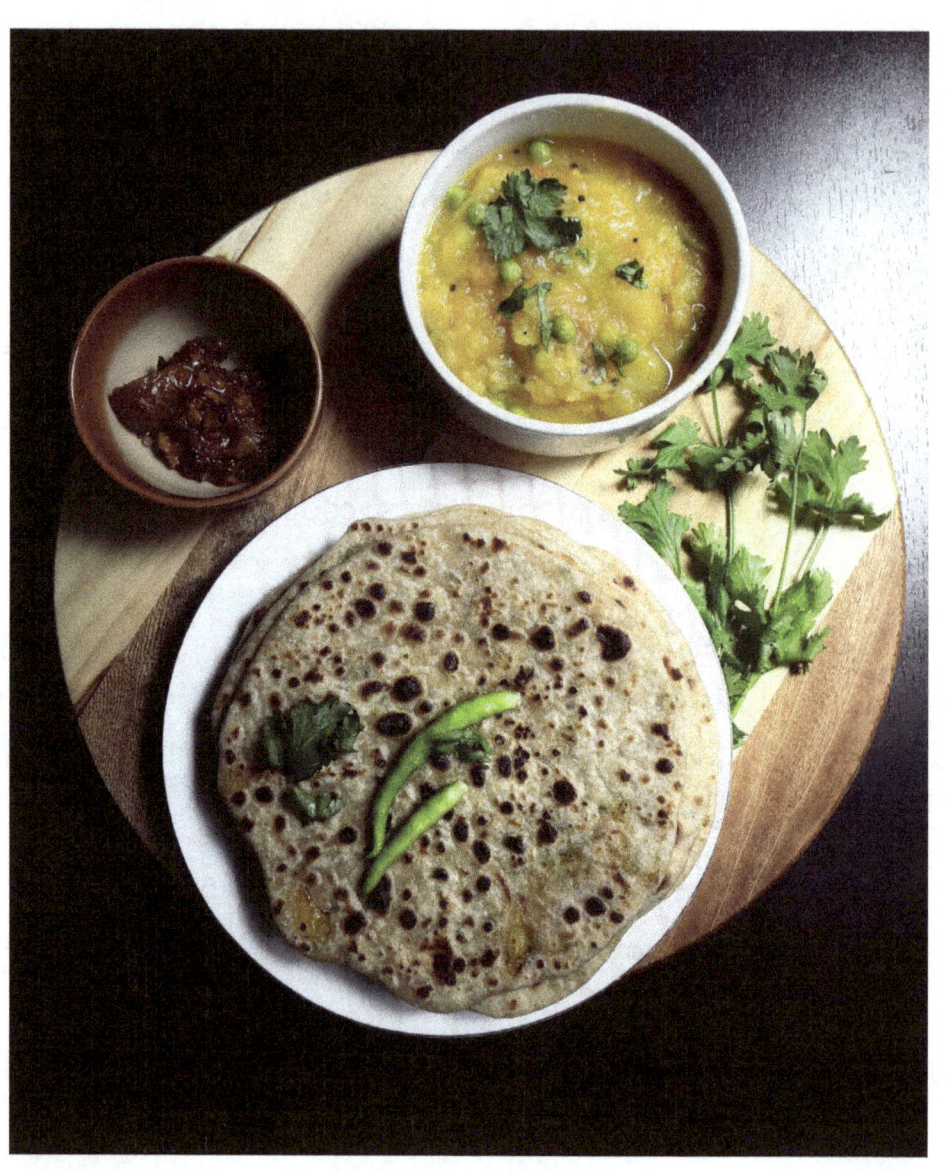

Orange Squares

Prep time: 2 hours I **Cooking time:** 0 minutes I
Servings: 4

Ingredients:

- 1/3 cup natural coconut butter, melted
- 1 and ½ tablespoons avocado oil
- 2 tablespoons orange juice
- ½ teaspoon orange zest, grated
- 1 tablespoons honey

Directions:

1. In a bowl, combine the coconut butter with the oil and the other ingredients, stir well, scoop into a square pan, spread well, cut into squares, keep in the freezer for 2 hours and serve.

Nutrition info per serving: calories 72, fat 4, fiber 2, carbs 8, protein 6

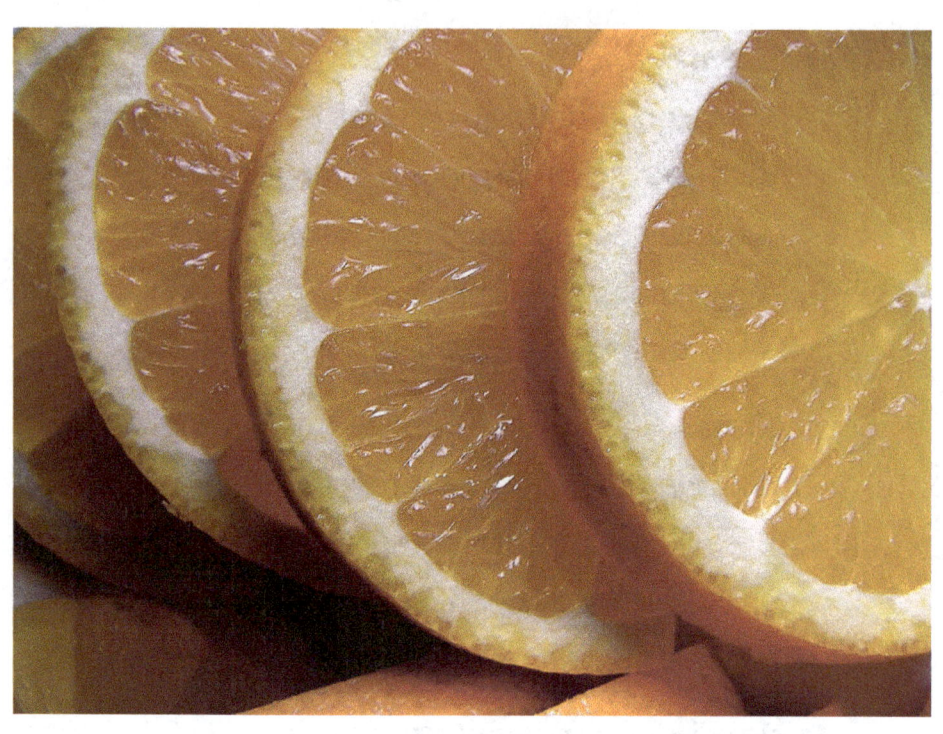

Chia and Honey Mix

Prep time: 10 minutes I **Cooking time:** 0 minutes I
Servings: 4

Ingredients:

- ¼ cup chia seeds
- 1 cup almond milk
- 2 mangos, peeled and cubed
- 2 teaspoons vanilla extract
- ¼ cup coconut, shredded
- 1 tablespoon honey

Directions:

1. In a bowl, combine the chia seeds with the mango, the milk and the other ingredients, toss, leave aside for 10 minutes, divide into small bowls and serve.

Nutrition info per serving: calories 287, fat 17.2, fiber 5.1, carbs 34.6, protein 3.2

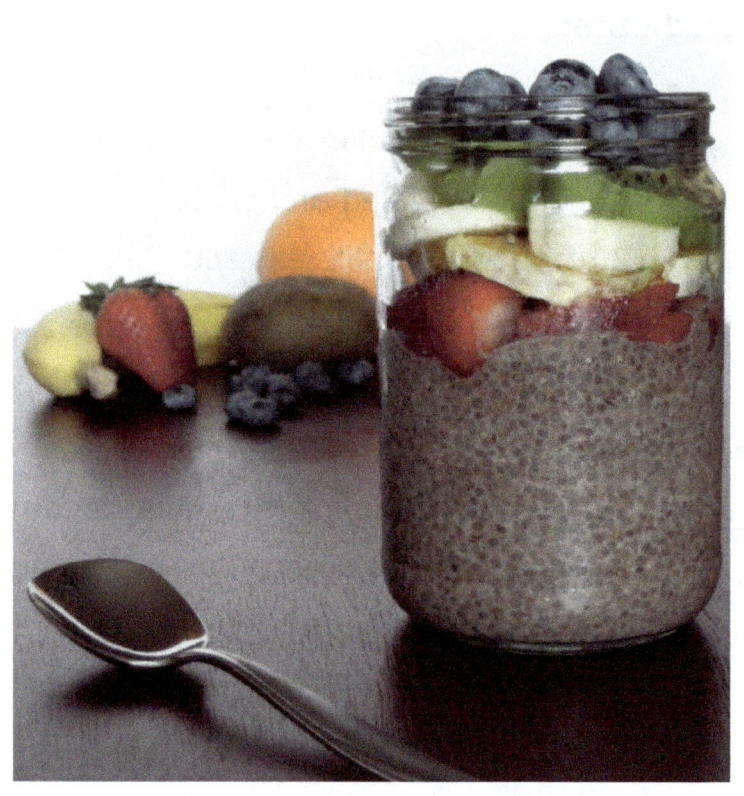

Pomegranate and Berries Mix

Prep time: 2 hours I **Cooking time:** 0 minutes I
Servings: 4

Ingredients:

- ½ cup coconut cream
- 1 orange, peeled and cut into wedges
- 1 teaspoon vanilla extract
- ½ cup almonds, chopped
- 1 cup pomegranate seeds
- 1 tablespoon orange zest, grated

Directions:

1. In a bowl, combine the orange with the pomegranate seeds and the other ingredients, toss and keep in the fridge for 2 hours before dividing into smaller bowls and serving.

Nutrition info per serving: calories 68, fat 5.1, fiber 4, carbs 6, protein 1

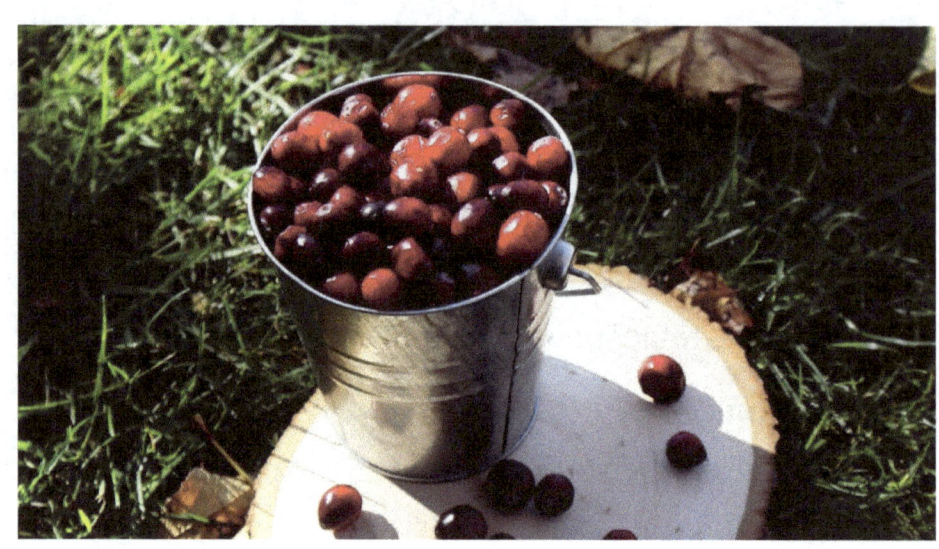

Almond Bowls

Prep time: 10 minutes

Cooking time: 0 minutes

Servings: 4

Ingredients:

- ½ teaspoon vanilla extract
- 1 cup almonds, chopped
- 1 tablespoon maple syrup
- 1 tablespoon coconut oil, melted

Directions:

1. In a bowl, combine the almonds and the other ingredients, toss, divide into small cups and serve.

Nutrition info per serving: calories 130, fat 5, fiber 5, carbs 12, protein 4

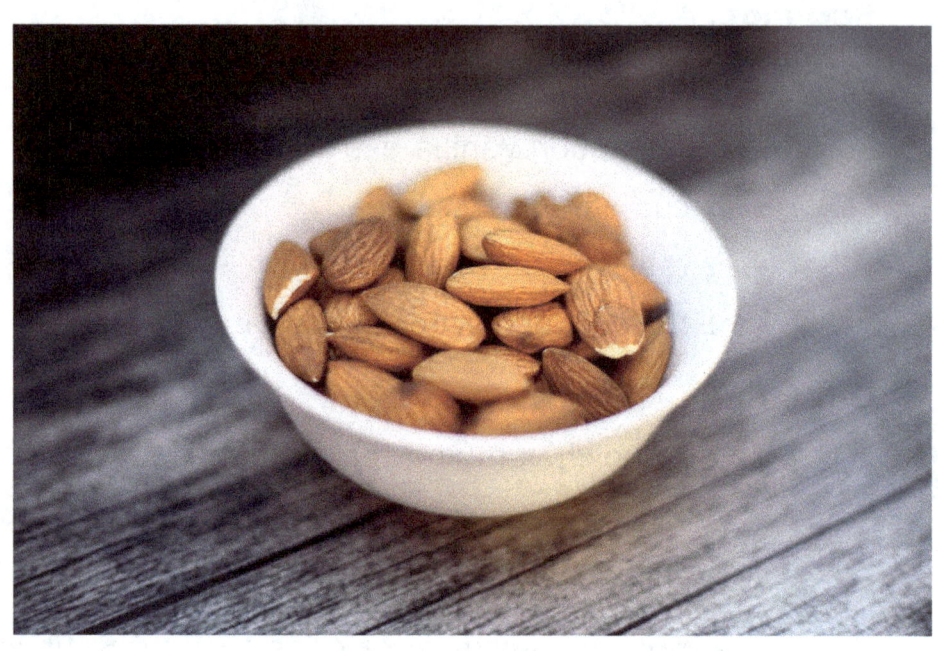

Apple Mint Cream

Prep time: 10 minutes I **Cooking time:** 0 minutes I
Servings: 4

Ingredients:

- 1 pounds apples, peeled, cored and cubed
- 2 cups coconut cream
- 1 tablespoon mint, chopped

Directions:

1. In your blender, combine the apples with the cream and mint, pulse well, divide into small cups and serve cold.

Nutrition info per serving: calories 70, fat 9, fiber 3, carbs 4.4, protein 3

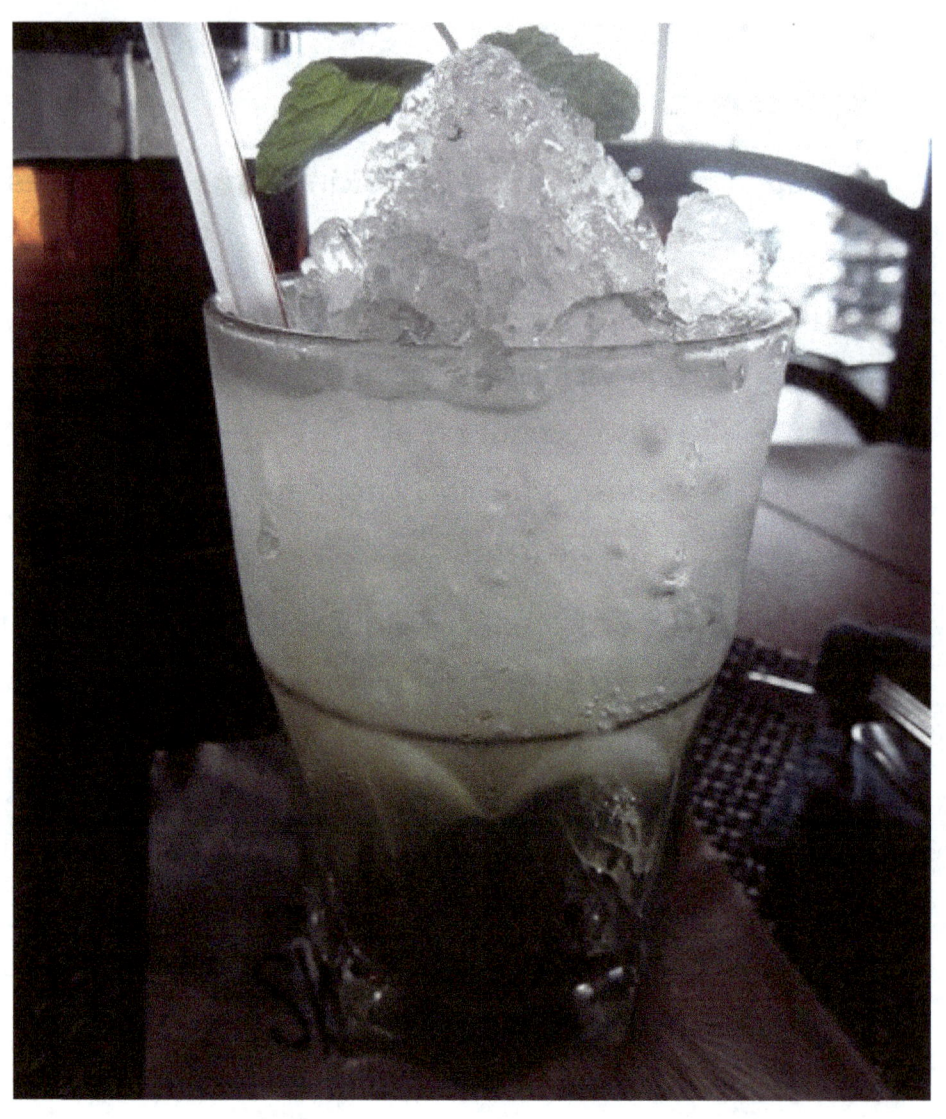

Cashews Bowls

Prep time: 10 minutes I **Cooking time:** 0 minutes I
Servings: 4

Ingredients:

- 1 cup cashews
- 2 cups blackberries
- ¾ cup coconut cream
- 1 teaspoon vanilla extract
- 1 tablespoon coconut sugar

Directions:

1. In a bowl, combine the cashews with the berries and the other ingredients, toss, divide into small bowls and serve.

Nutrition info per serving: calories 230, fat 4, fiber 3.4, carbs 12.3, protein 8

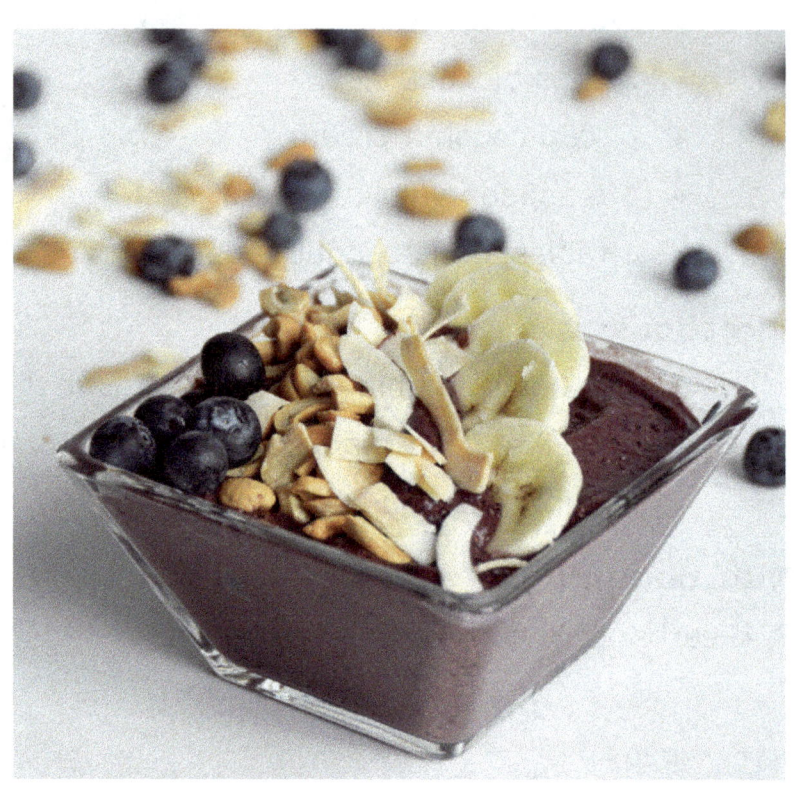

Orange Bowls

Prep time: 4 minutes I **Cooking time:** 8 minutes I
Servings: 4

Ingredients:

- 4 oranges, peeled and cut into segments
- Juice of 1 lime
- 2 tablespoons coconut sugar
- 1 cup water

Directions:

1. In a pan, combine the oranges and the other ingredients, bring to a simmer and cook over medium heat for 8 minutes.
2. Divide into bowls and serve cold.

Nutrition info per serving: calories 170, fat 2.3, fiber 2.3, carbs 11, protein 3.4

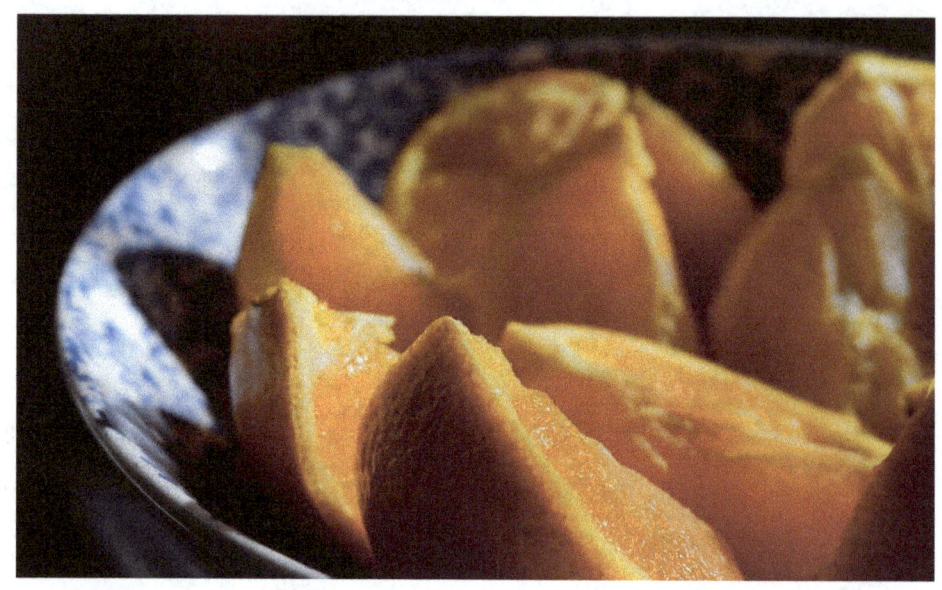

Pumpkin Cream

Prep time: 2 hours I **Cooking time:** 0 minutes I
Servings: 4

Ingredients:

- 2 cups coconut cream
- 1 cup pumpkin puree
- 14 ounces coconut cream
- 3 tablespoons coconut sugar

Directions:

1. In a bowl, combine the cream with the pumpkin puree and the other ingredients, whisk well, divide into small bowls and keep in the fridge for 2 hours before serving.

Nutrition info per serving: calories 350, fat 12.3, fiber 3, carbs 11.7, protein 6

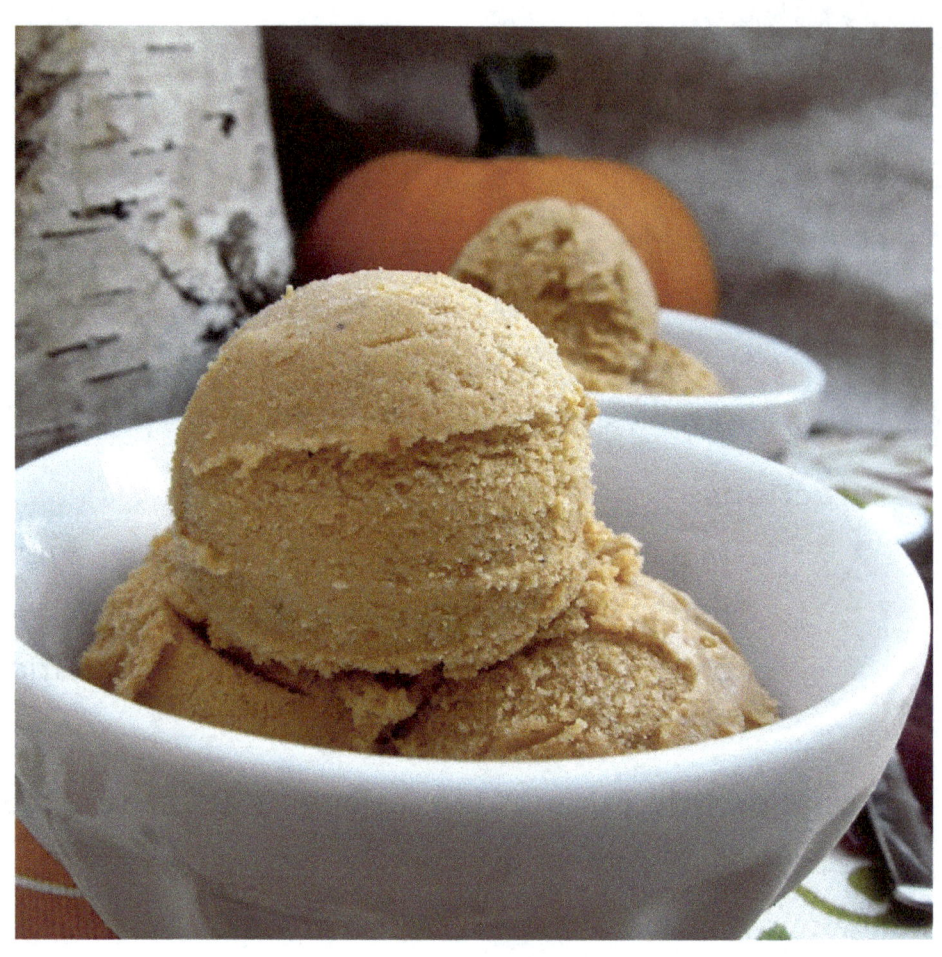

Figs Mix

Prep time: 6 minutes I **Cooking time:** 14 minutes I
Servings: 4

Ingredients:

- 2 tablespoons avocado oil
- 1 teaspoon vanilla extract
- 12 figs, halved
- ¼ cup coconut sugar
- 1 cup water

Directions:

1. Heat up a pan with the oil over medium heat, add the figs and the rest of the ingredients, toss, cook for 14 minutes, divide into small cups and serve cold.

Nutrition info per serving: calories 213, fat 7.4, fiber 6.1, carbs 39, protein 2.2

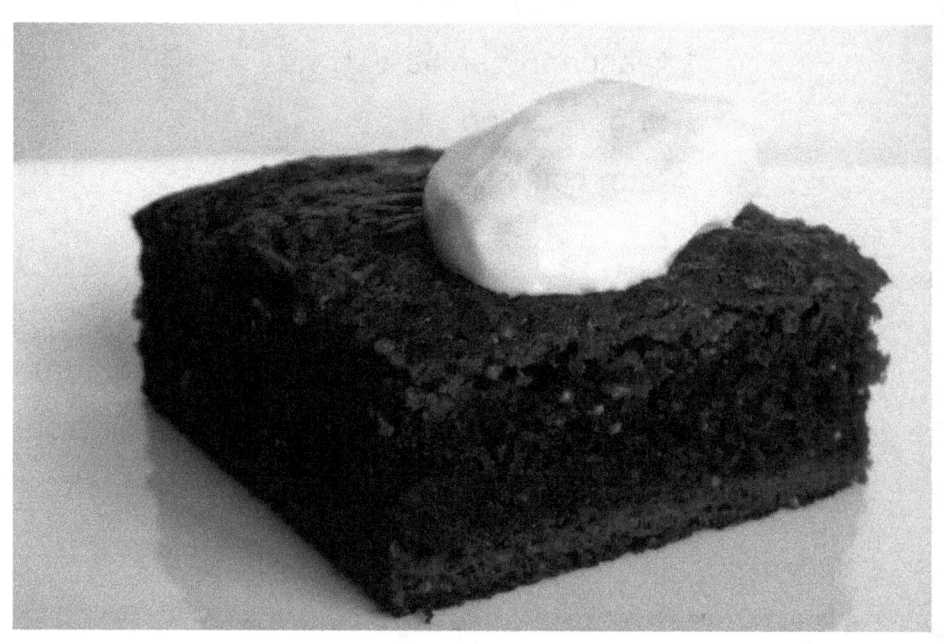

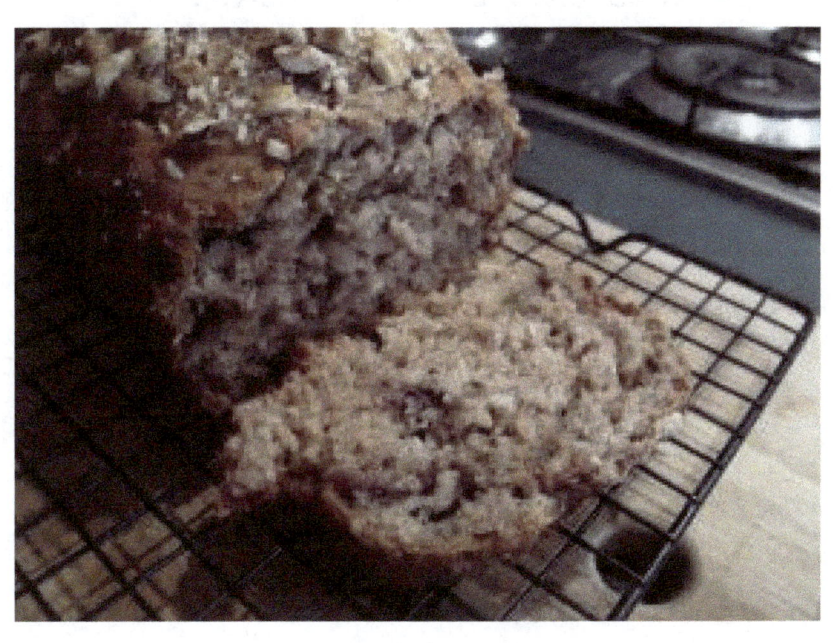

Nutmeg Banana

Prep time: 4 minutes I **Cooking time:** 15 minutes I
Servings: 4

Ingredients:

- 4 bananas, peeled and halved
- 1 teaspoon nutmeg, ground
- 1 teaspoon cinnamon powder
- Juice of 1 lime
- 4 tablespoons coconut sugar

Directions:

1. Arrange the bananas in a baking pan, add the nutmeg and the other ingredients, bake at 350 degrees F for 15 minutes.
2. Divide the baked bananas between plates and serve.

Nutrition info per serving: calories 206, fat 0.6, fiber 3.2, carbs 47.1, protein 2.4

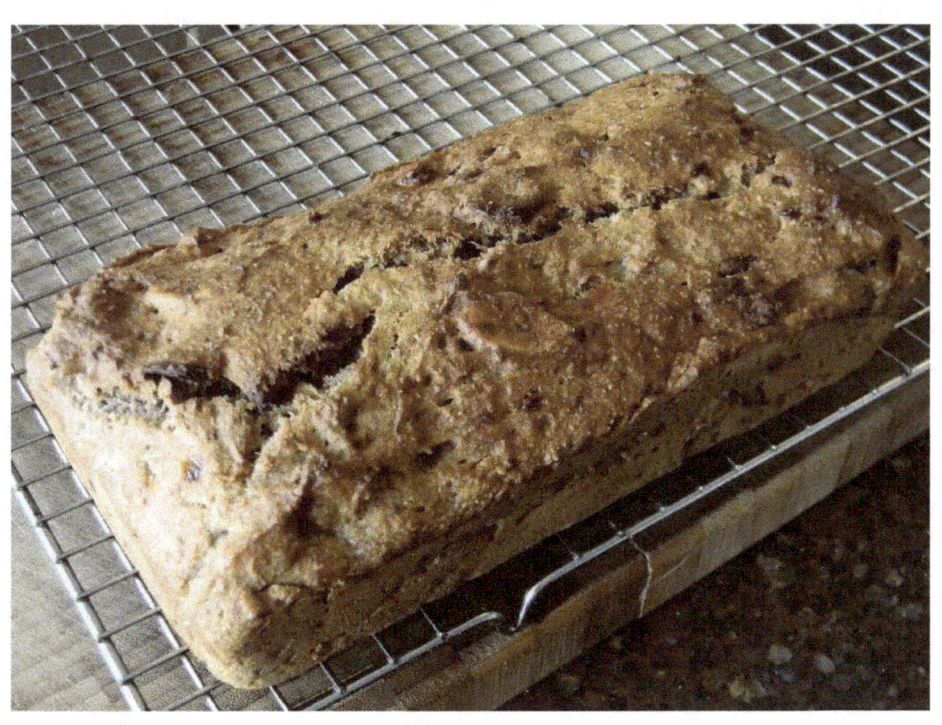

Cocoa Smoothie

Prep time: 5 minutes I **Cooking time:** 0 minutes I
Servings: 2

Ingredients:

- 2 teaspoons cocoa powder
- 1 avocado, pitted, peeled and mashed
- 1 cup almond milk
- 1 cup coconut cream

Directions:

1. In your blender, combine the almond milk with the cream and the other ingredients, pulse well, divide in to cups and serve cold.

Nutrition info per serving: calories 155, fat 12.3, fiber 4, carbs 8.6, protein 5

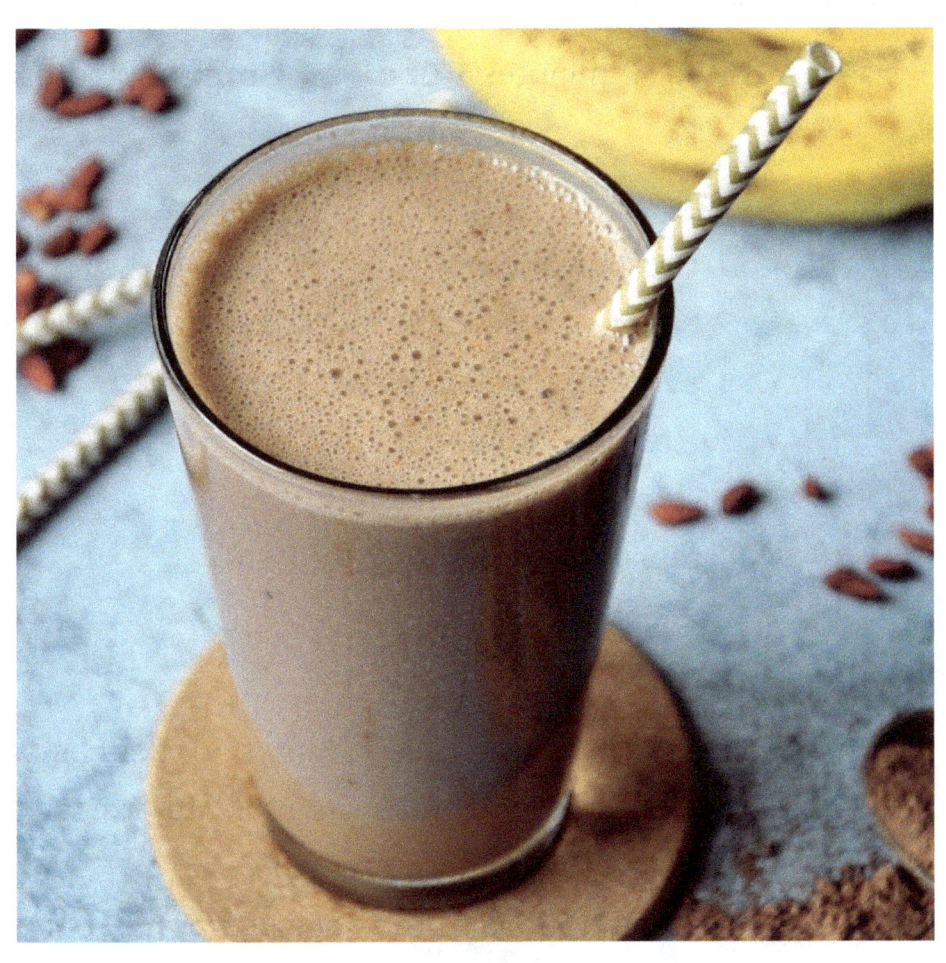

Banana Bars

Prep time: 30 minutes I **Cooking time:** 0 minutes I
Servings: 4

Ingredients:

- 1 cup avocado oil
- 2 bananas, peeled and chopped
- 1 avocado, peeled, pitted and mashed
- ½ cup coconut sugar
- ¼ cup lime juice
- 1 teaspoon lemon zest, grated
- Cooking spray

Directions:

1. In your food processor, mix the bananas with the oil and the other ingredients except the cooking spray and pulse well.
2. Grease a pan with the cooking spray, pour and spread the banana mix, spread, keep in the fridge for 30 minutes, cut into bars and serve.

Nutrition info per serving: calories 639, fat 64.6, fiber 4.9, carbs 20.5, protein 1.7

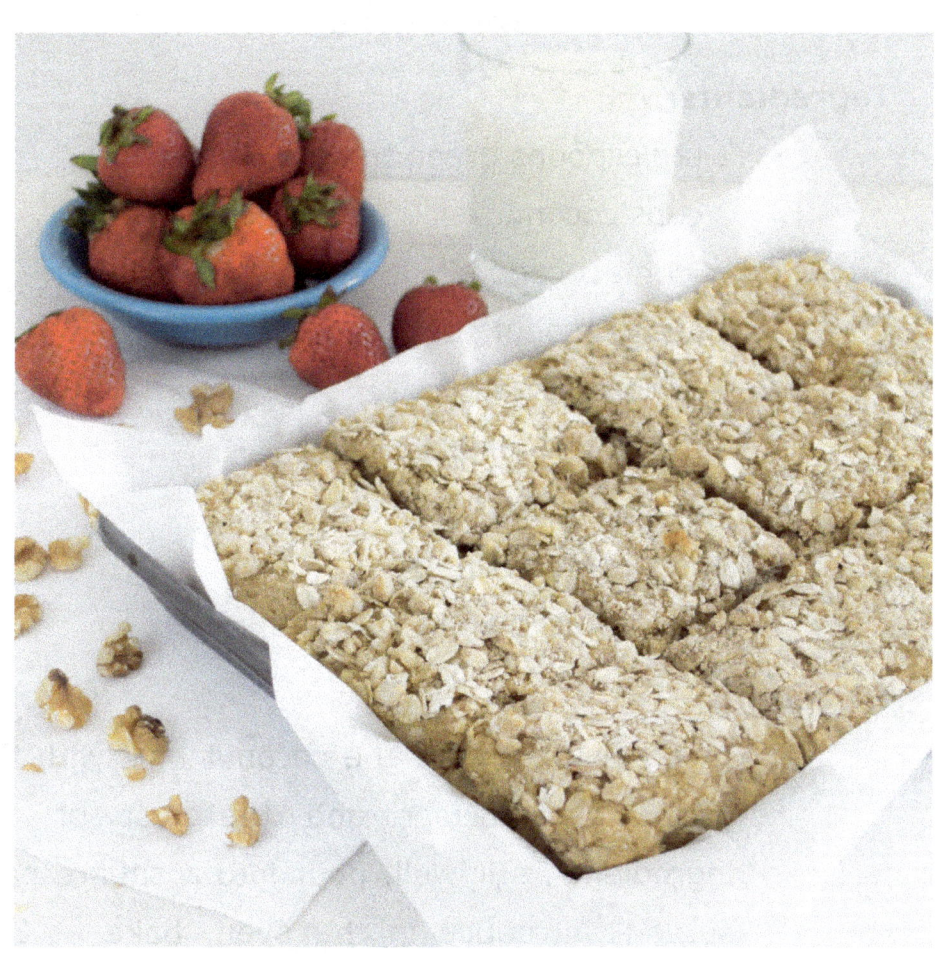

Green Tea Bars

Prep time: 10 minutes I **Cooking time:** 30 minutes I **Servings:** 8

Ingredients:

- 2 tablespoons green tea powder
- 2 cups coconut milk, heated
- ½ cup avocado oil
- 2 cups coconut sugar
- 4 eggs, whisked
- 2 teaspoons vanilla extract
- 3 cups almond flour
- 1 teaspoon baking soda
- 2 teaspoons baking powder

Directions:

1. In a bowl, combine the coconut milk with the green tea powder and the rest of the ingredients, stir well, pour into a square pan, spread, introduce in the oven, bake at 350 degrees F for 30 minutes, cool down, cut into bars and serve.

Nutrition info per serving: calories 560, fat 22.3, fiber 4, carbs 12.8, protein 22.1

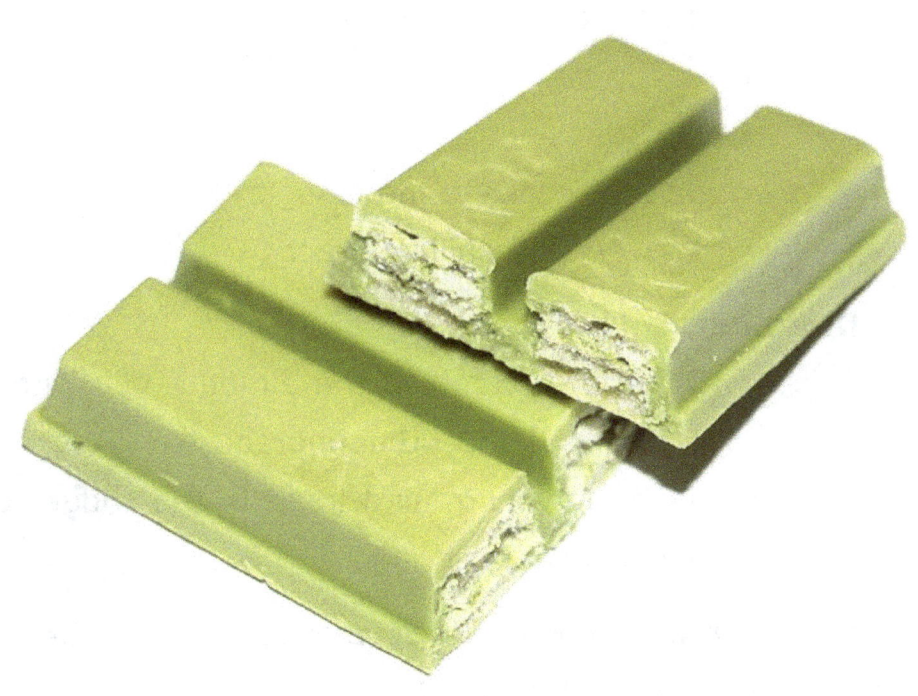

Walnut Cream

Prep time: 2 hours I **Cooking time:** 0 minutes I
Servings: 4

Ingredients:

- 2 cups almond milk
- ½ cup coconut cream
- ½ cup walnuts, chopped
- 3 tablespoons coconut sugar
- 1 teaspoon vanilla extract

Directions:

1. In a bowl, combine the almond milk with the cream and the other ingredients, whisk well, divide into cups and keep in the fridge for 2 hours before serving.

Nutrition info per serving: calories 170, fat 12.4, fiber 3, carbs 12.8, protein 4

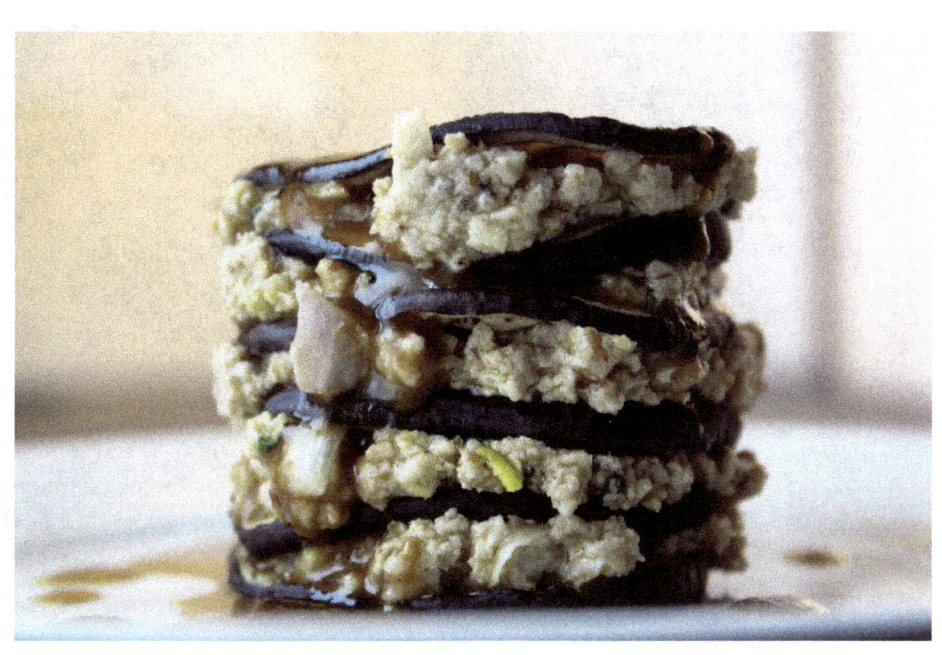

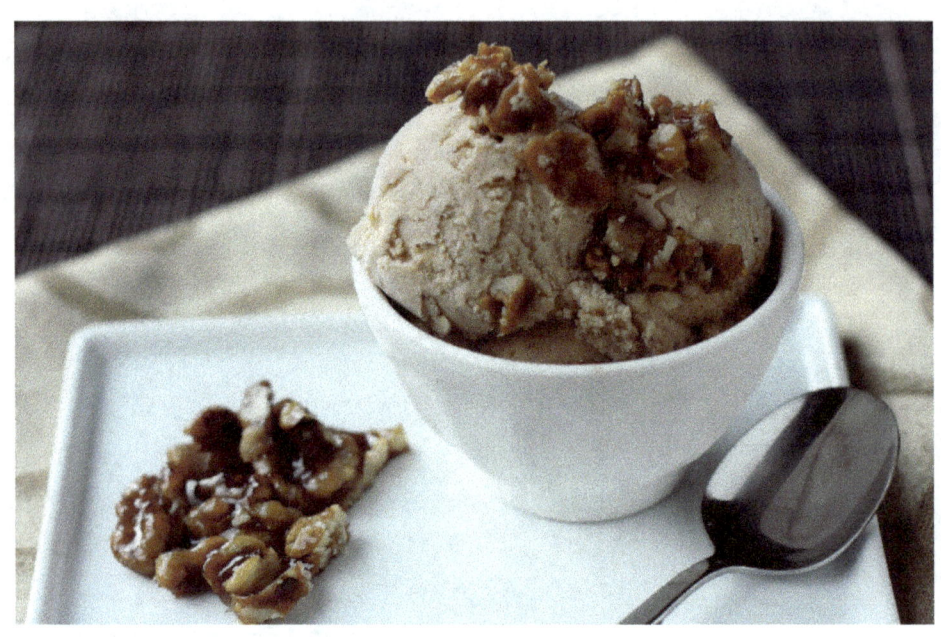

Lemon Almond Cake

Prep time: 10 minutes I **Cooking time:** 35 minutes I
Servings: 6

Ingredients:

- 2 cups almond flour
- 1 teaspoon baking powder
- 2 tablespoons avocado oil
- 1 egg, whisked
- 3 tablespoons coconut sugar
- 1 cup almond milk
- Zest of 1 lemon, grated
- Juice of 1 lemon

Directions:

1. In a bowl, combine the flour with the oil and the other ingredients, whisk well, transfer this to a cake pan and bake at 360 degrees F for 35 minutes.
2. Slice and serve cold.

Nutrition info per serving: calories 222, fat 12.5, fiber 6.2, carbs 7, protein 17.4

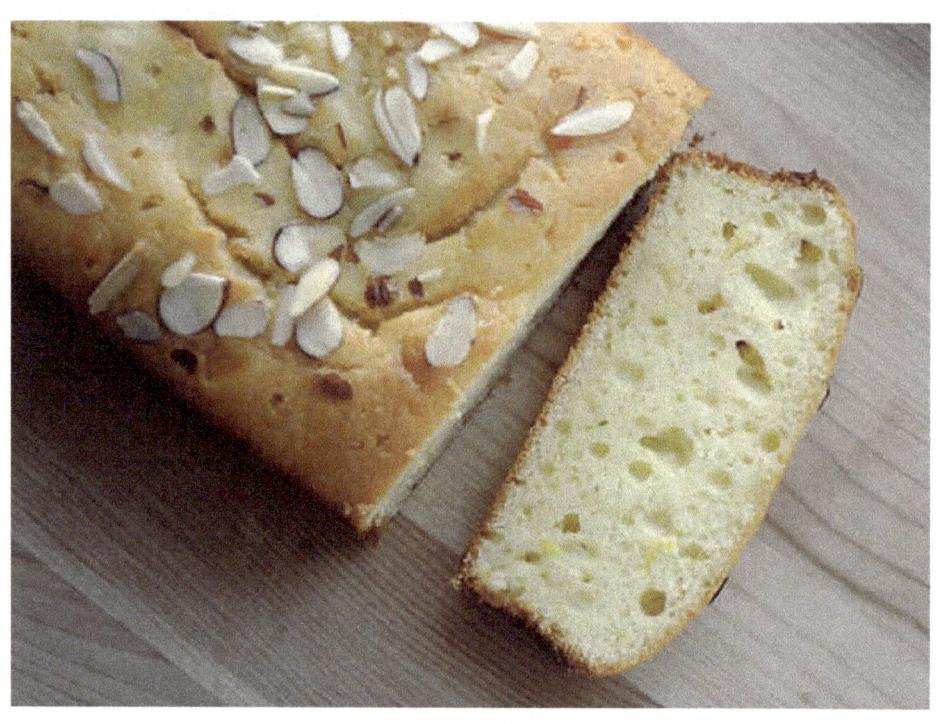

Nutmeg Raisins Bars

Prep time: 10 minutes I **Cooking time:** 25 minutes I
Servings: 6

Ingredients:

- 1 teaspoon cinnamon powder
- 2 cups almond flour
- 1 teaspoon baking powder
- ½ teaspoon nutmeg, ground
- 1 cup avocado oil
- 1 cup coconut sugar
- 1 egg, whisked
- 1 cup raisins

Directions:

1. In a bowl, combine the flour with the cinnamon and the other ingredients, stir well, spread on a lined baking sheet, introduce in the oven, bake at 380 degrees F for 25 minutes, cut into bars and serve cold.

Nutrition info per serving: calories 274, fat 12, fiber 5.2, carbs 14.5, protein 7

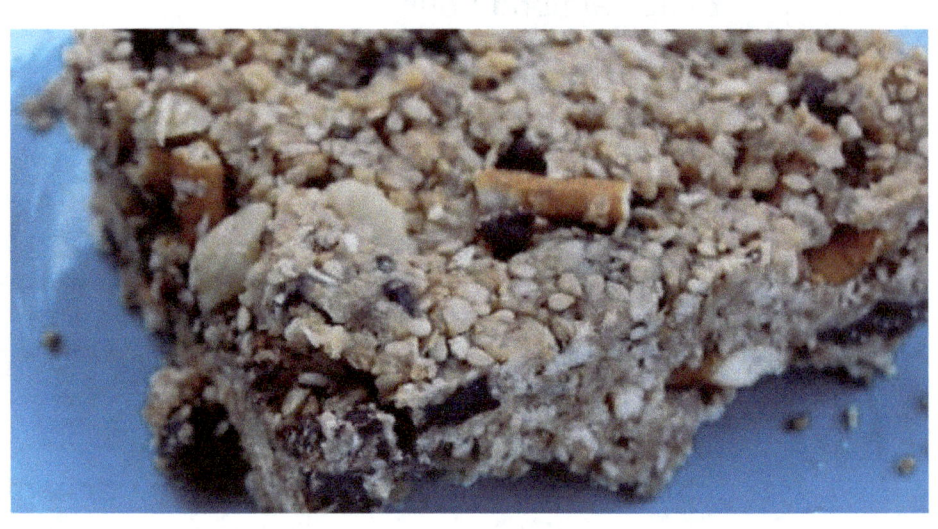

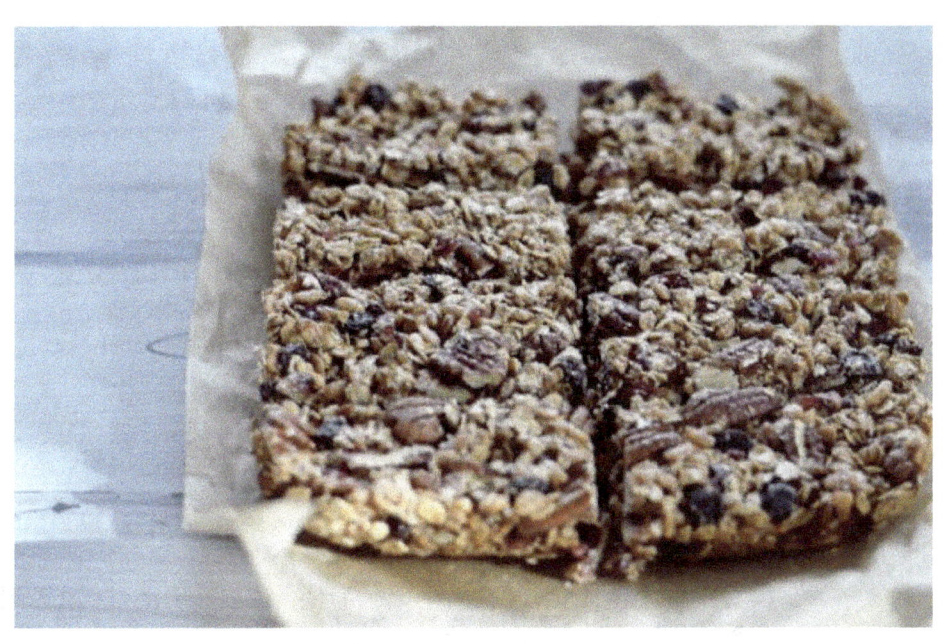

Citrus Squares

Prep time: 10 minutes I **Cooking time:** 20 minutes I
Servings: 4

Ingredients:

- 3 nectarines, pitted and chopped
- 1 tablespoon coconut sugar
- ½ teaspoon baking soda
- 1 cup almond flour
- 4 tablespoons avocado oil
- 2 tablespoons cocoa powder

Directions:

1. In a blender, combine the nectarines with the sugar and the rest of the ingredients, pulse well, pour into a lined square pan, spread, bake in the oven at 375 degrees F for 20 minutes, leave the mix aside to cool down a bit, cut into squares and serve.

Nutrition info per serving: calories 342, fat 14.4, fiber 7.6, carbs 12, protein 7.7

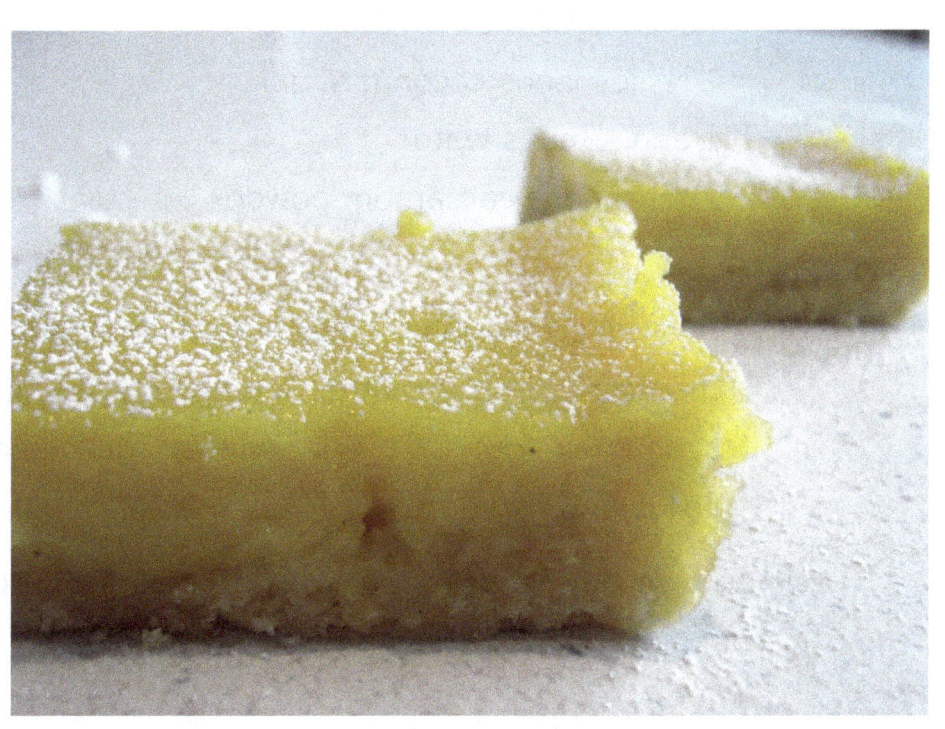

Lime Grapes Stew

Prep time: 10 minutes I **Cooking time:** 20 minutes I
Servings: 4

Ingredients:

- 1 cup green grapes
- Juice of ½ lime
- 2 tablespoons coconut sugar
- 1 and ½ cups water
- 2 teaspoons cardamom powder

Directions:

1. Heat up a pan with the water medium heat, add the grapes and the other ingredients, bring to a simmer, cook for 20 minutes, divide into bowls and serve.

Nutrition info per serving: calories 384, fat 12.5, fiber 6.3, carbs 13.8, protein 5.6

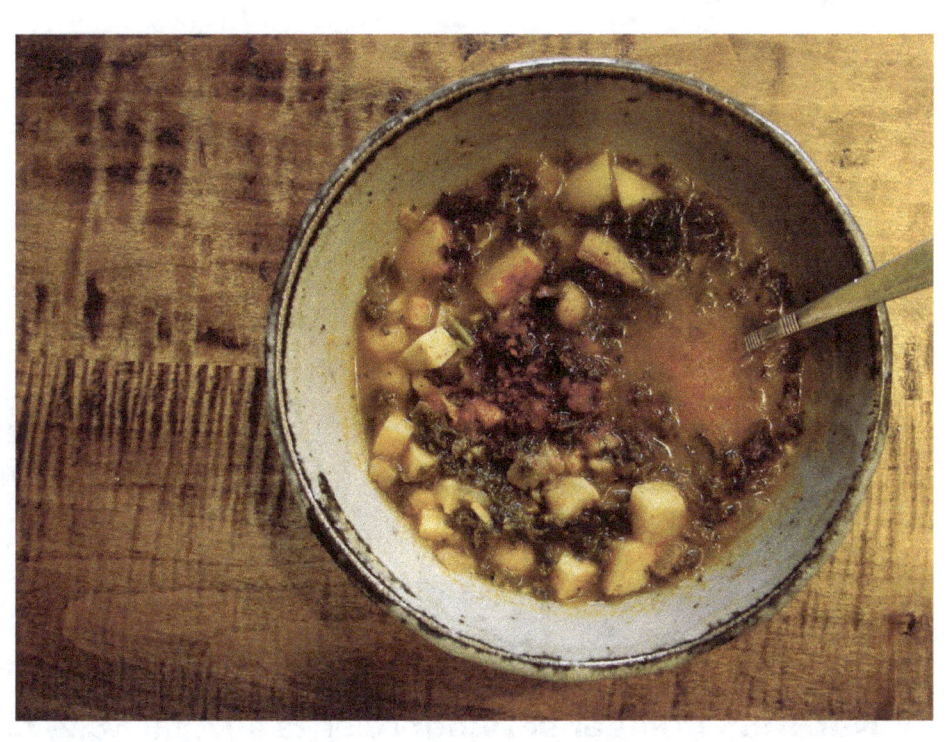

Mandarin Cream

Prep time: 10 minutes I **Cooking time:** 20 minutes I
Servings: 4

Ingredients:

- 1 mandarin, peeled and chopped
- ½ pound plums, pitted and chopped
- 1 cup coconut cream
- Juice of 2 mandarins
- 2 tablespoons coconut sugar

Directions:

1. In a blender, combine the mandarin with the plums and the other ingredients, pulse well, divide into small ramekins, introduce in the oven, bake at 350 degrees F for 20 minutes, and serve cold.

Nutrition info per serving: calories 402, fat 18.2, fiber 2, carbs 22.2, protein 4.5

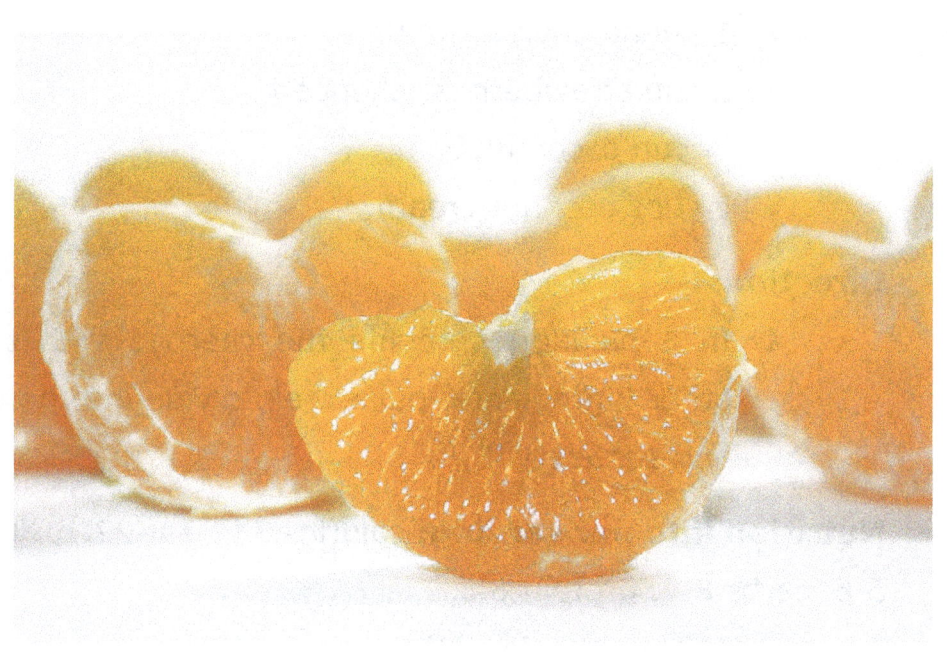

Cherry Cream

Prep time: 10 minutes I **Cooking time:** 0 minutes I
Servings: 6

Ingredients:

- 1 pound cherries, pitted
- 1 cup strawberries, chopped
- ¼ cup coconut sugar
- 2 cups coconut cream

Directions:

1. In a blender, combine the cherries with the other ingredients, pulse well, divide into bowls and serve cold.

Nutrition info per serving: calories 342, fat 22.1, fiber 5.6, carbs 8.4, protein 6.5

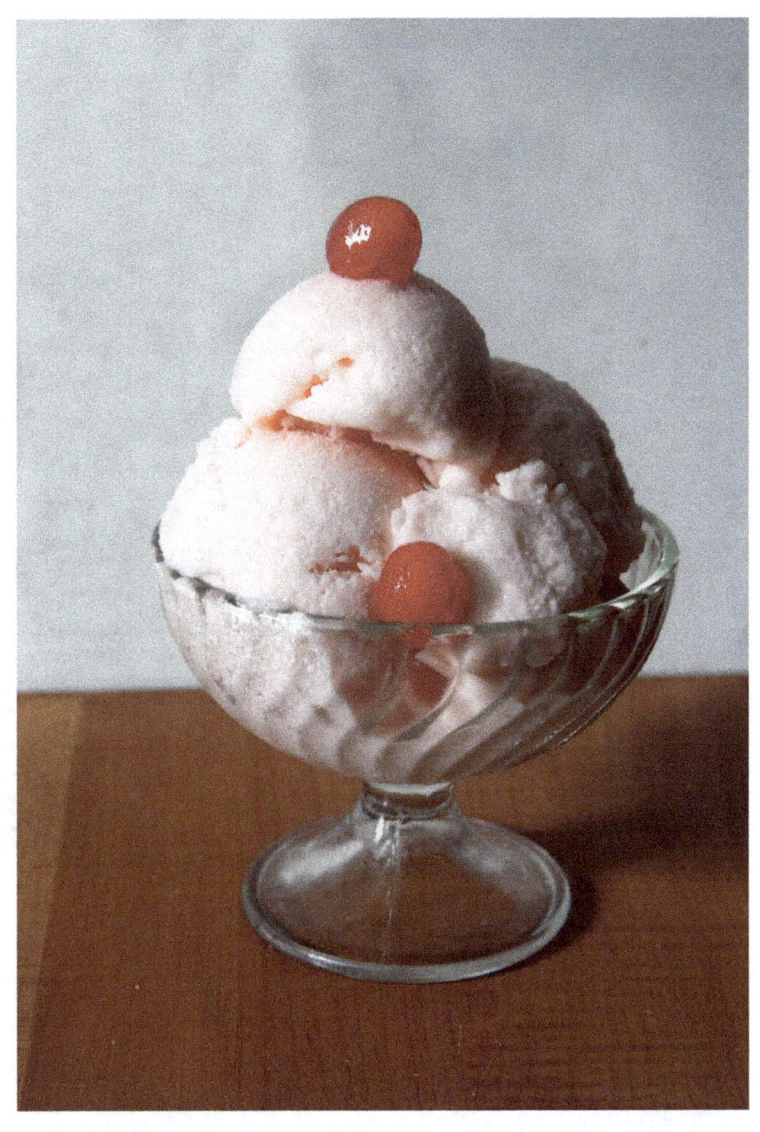

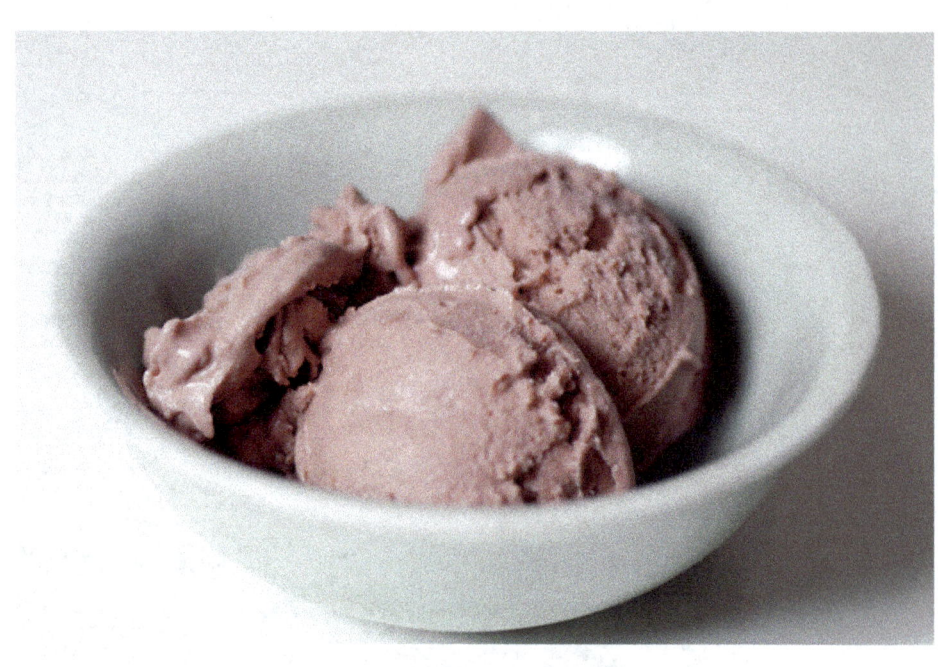

Cardamom Pudding

Prep time: 5 minutes I **Cooking time:** 40 minutes I
Servings: 4

Ingredients:

- 1 cup brown rice
- 3 cups almond milk
- 3 tablespoons coconut sugar
- ½ teaspoon cardamom powder
- ¼ cup walnuts, chopped

Directions:

1. In a pan, combine the brown rice with the milk and the other ingredients, stir, cook for 40 minutes over medium heat, divide into bowls and serve cold.

Nutrition info per serving: calories 703, fat 47.9, fiber 5.2, carbs 62.1, protein 10.1

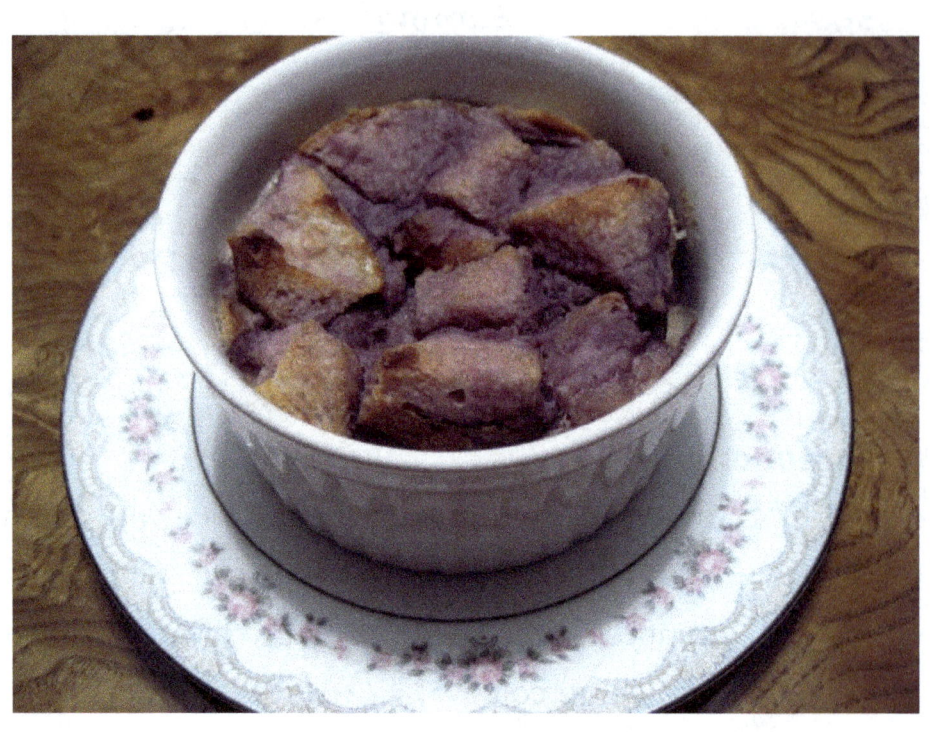

Fruity Bread

Prep time: 10 minutes I **Cooking time:** 30 minutes I
Servings: 4

Ingredients:

- 2 cups pears, cored and cubed
- 1 cup coconut sugar
- 2 eggs, whisked
- 2 cups almond flour
- 1 tablespoon baking powder
- 1 tablespoon coconut oil, melted

Directions:

1. In a bowl, mix the pears with the sugar and the
   other ingredients, whisk, pour into a loaf pan,
   introduce in the oven and bake at 350 degrees
   F for 30 minutes.
2. Slice and serve cold.

Nutrition info per serving: calories 380, fat 16.7, fiber
5, carbs 17.5, protein 5.6

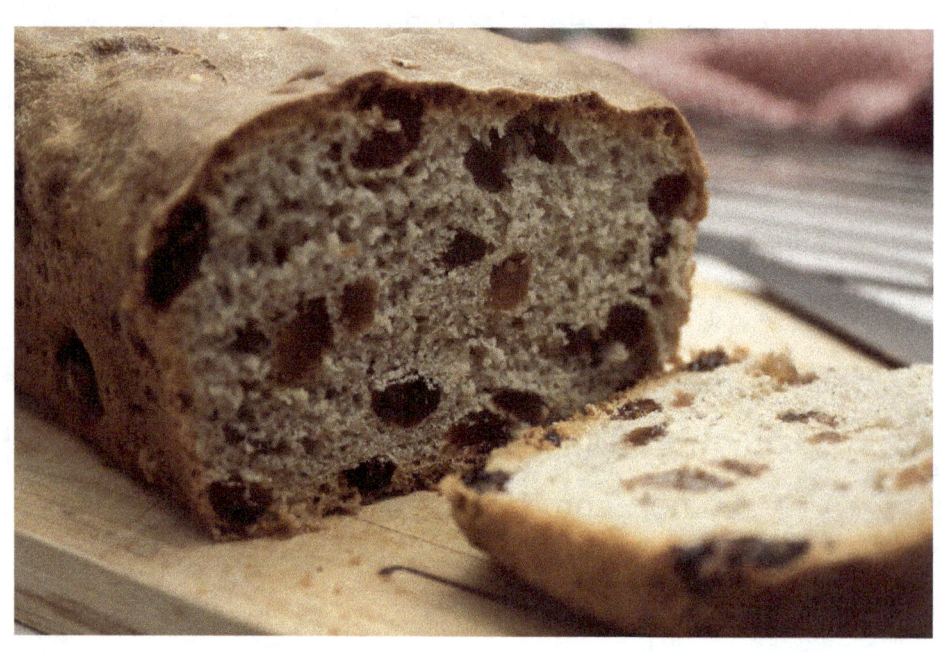

Rice Almond Pudding

Prep time: 10 minutes I **Cooking time:** 25 minutes I
Servings: 4

Ingredients:

- 1 tablespoon avocado oil
- 1 cup brown rice
- 3 cups almond milk
- ½ cup cherries, pitted and halved
- 3 tablespoons coconut sugar
- 1 teaspoon cinnamon powder
- 1 teaspoon vanilla extract

Directions:

1. In a pan, combine the oil with the rice and the other ingredients, stir, bring to a simmer, cook for 25 minutes over medium heat, divide into bowls and serve cold.

Nutrition info per serving: calories 292, fat 12.4, fiber 5.6, carbs 8, protein 7

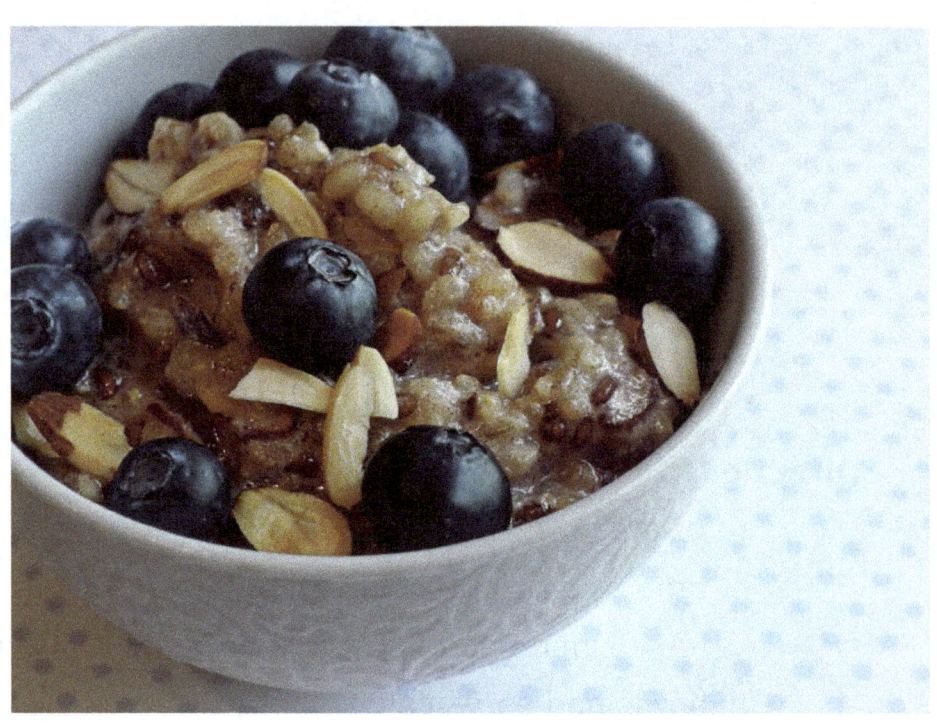

Watermelon Stew

Prep time: 5 minutes I **Cooking time:** 8 minutes I
Servings: 4

Ingredients:

- Juice of 1 lime
- 1 teaspoon lime zest, grated
- 1 and ½ cup coconut sugar
- 4 cups watermelon, peeled and cut into large chunks
- 1 and ½ cups water

Directions:

1. In a pan, combine the watermelon with the lime zest, and the other ingredients, toss, bring to a simmer over medium heat, cook for 8 minutes, divide into bowls and serve cold.

Nutrition info per serving: calories 233, fat 0.2, fiber 0.7, carbs 61.5, protein 0.9

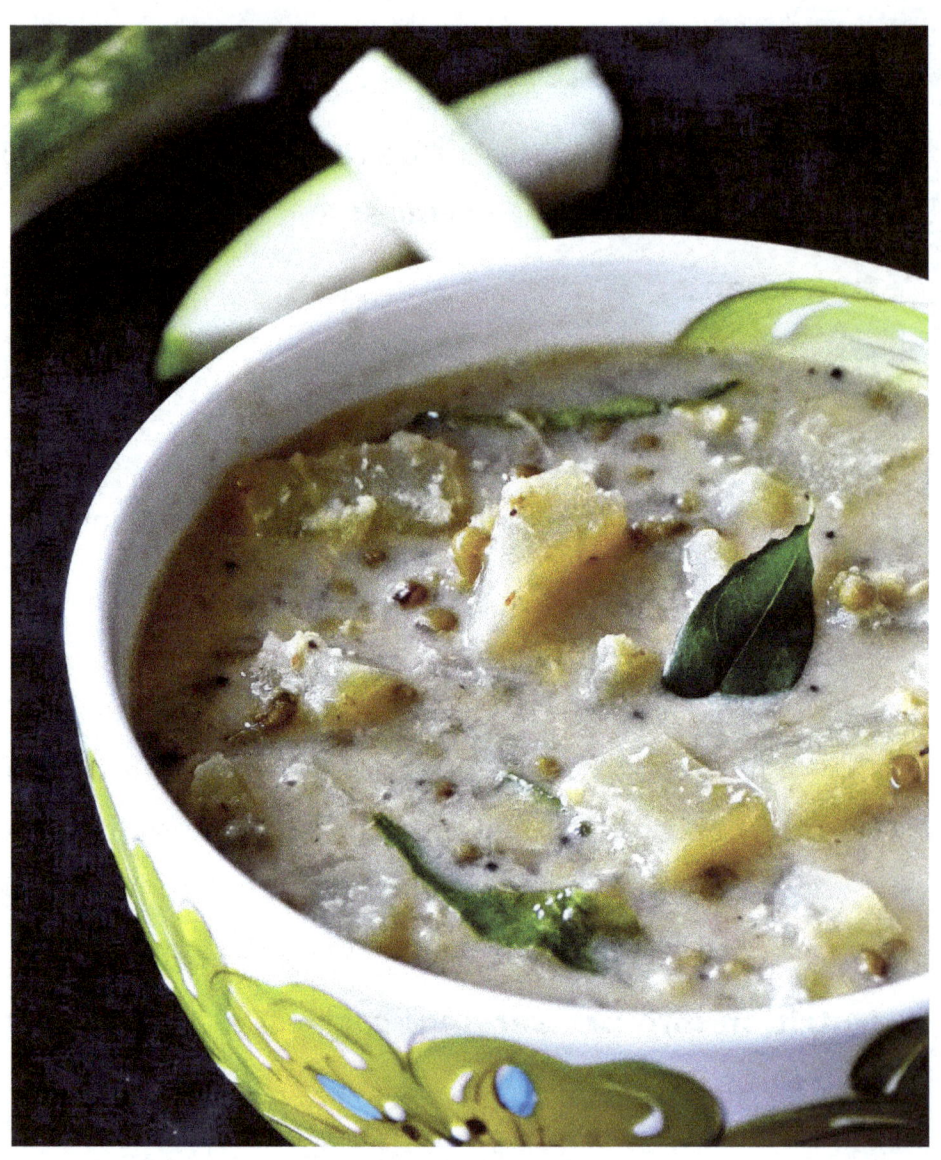

Ginger Chia Pudding

Prep time: 1 hour I **Cooking time:** 0 minutes I
Servings: 4

Ingredients:

- 2 cups almond milk
- ½ cup coconut cream
- 2 tablespoons coconut sugar
- 1 tablespoon ginger, grated
- ¼ cup chia seeds

Directions:

1. In a bowl, combine the milk with the cream and the other ingredients, whisk well, divide into small cups and keep them in the fridge for 1 hour before serving.

Nutrition info per serving: calories 345, fat 17, fiber 4.7, carbs 11.5, protein 6.9

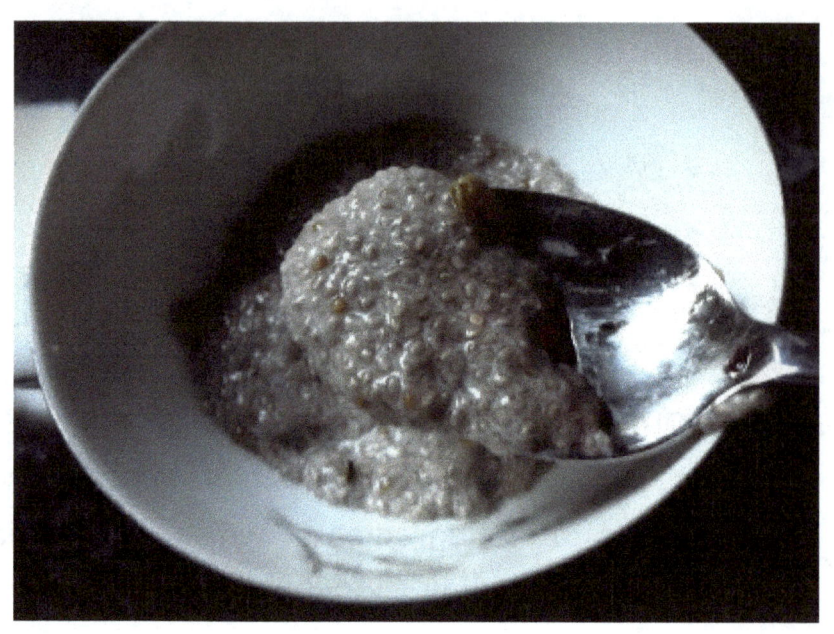

Cashew Cream

Prep time: 2 hours I **Cooking time:** 0 minutes I
Servings: 4

Ingredients:

- 1 cup cashews, chopped
- 2 tablespoons coconut oil, melted
- 2 tablespoons coconut oil, melted
- 1 cup coconut cream
- 2 tablespoons lemon juice
- 1 tablespoons coconut sugar

Directions:

1. In a blender, combine the cashews with the coconut oil and the other ingredients, pulse well, divide into small cups and keep in the fridge for 2 hours before serving.

Nutrition info per serving: calories 480, fat 43.9, fiber 2.4, carbs 19.7, protein 7

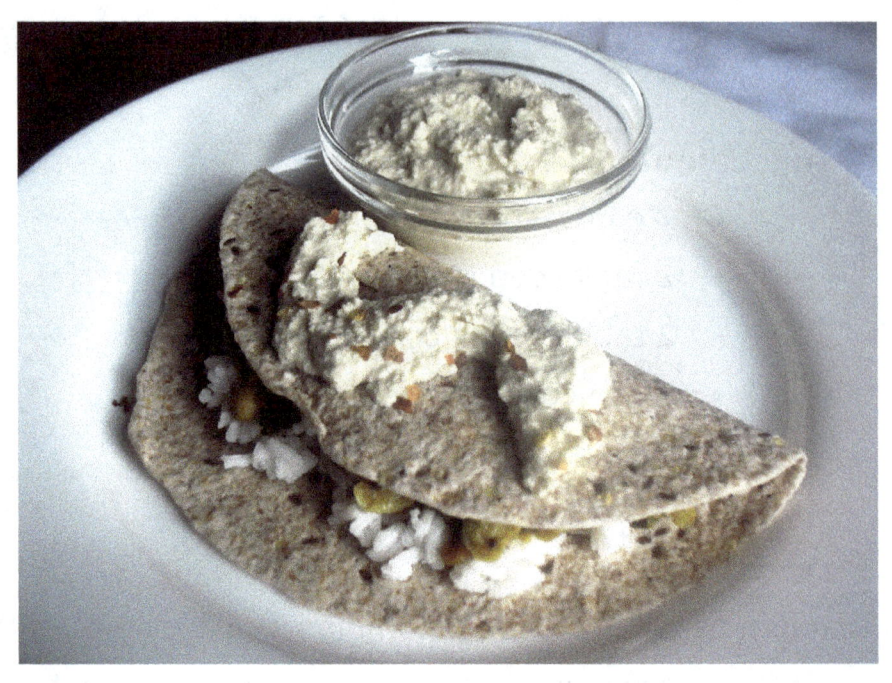